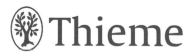

OCT Angiography

David R. Chow, MD, FRCSC
Assistant Professor
Department of Ophthalmology
St. Michaels Hospital
University of Toronto
Fellowship Director and Co-Director
Toronto Retina Institute
Toronto, Ontario, Canada

Paulo Ricardo Chaves de Oliveira, MD
Ophthalmology degree
Faculdade de Ciências Médicas da Santa Casa de São Paulo
Retinal Fellowship
Retina Clinic, São Paulo
Uveitis Fellowship
Federal University of São Paulo (UNIFESP)
Retinal Research Fellow
Toronto Retina Institute, Canada
Retinal Specialist
Instituto Panamericano da Visão
Goiânia, Brazil

Thieme
New York • Stuttgart • Delhi • Rio de Janeiro

Executive Editor: William Lamsback
Managing Editor: Haley Paskalides
Director, Editorial Services: Mary Jo Casey
Production Editor: Sean Woznicki
International Production Director: Andreas Schabert
Editorial Director: Sue Hodgson
International Marketing Director: Fiona Henderson
International Sales Director: Louisa Turrell
Director of Institutional Sales: Adam Bernacki
Senior Vice President and Chief Operating Officer:
Sarah Vanderbilt
President: Brian D. Scanlan

Library of Congress Cataloging-in-Publication Data

Names: Chow, David R., editor. | Oliveira, Paulo Ricardo
    Chaves de, editor.
Title: OCT angiography / [edited by] David R. Chow, Paulo
    Ricardo Chaves de Oliveira.
Description: New York, NY : Thieme Medical Publishers, Inc.,
    [2018] |
    Includes bibliographical references.
Identifiers: LCCN 2017032576| ISBN 9781626234734 (print) |
    ISBN 9781626234741 (e book)
Subjects: | MESH: Retinal Diseases–diagnostic imaging |
    Tomography, Optical Coherence | Computed Tomography
    Angiography | Eye Diseases–diagnostic imaging | Retinal
    Vessels–diagnostic imaging | Case Reports
Classification: LCC RE79.I42 | NLM WW 270 | DDC 616.07/545–
dc23 LC record available at https://lccn.loc.gov/2017032576

© 2018 Thieme Medical Publishers, Inc.

Thieme Publishers New York
333 Seventh Avenue, New York, NY 10001 USA
+1 800 782 3488, customerservice@thieme.com

Thieme Publishers Stuttgart
Rüdigerstrasse 14, 70469 Stuttgart, Germany
+49 [0]711 8931 421, customerservice@thieme.de

Thieme Publishers Delhi
A-12, Second Floor, Sector-2, Noida-201301
Uttar Pradesh, India
+91 120 45 566 00, customerservice@thieme.in

Thieme Publishers Rio de Janeiro, Thieme Publicações Ltda.
Edifício Rodolpho de Paoli, 25º andar
Av. Nilo Peçanha, 50 – Sala 2508,
Rio de Janeiro 20020-906 Brasil
+55 21 3172-2297 / +55 21 3172-1896

Cover design: Thieme Publishing Group
Typesetting by Thomson Digital, India

Printed in the United States of America by,   5 4 3 2
King Printing Co., Inc.

ISBN 978-1-62623-473-4

Also available as an e-book:
eISBN 978-1-62623-474-1

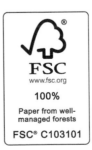

Any significant effort or venture requires a lot of help to do properly. This textbook was no different. I would like to thank the authors who provide authoritative views on their areas of expertise and do so for only academic and educational reasons. Paulo Oliveira was my research fellow from Brazil who helped me get this done. It would not have happened without him. Thanks Paulo! And to my family who see me running all over the place. Don't forget you are all more important to me than anything I do at work.

Contents

Contents

Contents

Preface

Ophthalmologists are fortunate to be the recipient of great advances in technology. Over and over, we are presented with exciting new technologies to aid in the diagnosis of our patients and to treat our patients in the office or operating room. Without question one of the areas that will change the most over the next decade will be imaging technologies that will make the examining room of the 21st-century retina specialist a very technologically savvy thing! Optical coherence tomography (OCT) angiography will be one of the exciting new imaging technologies that will transform our office. It offers ophthalmologists the ability to image the vasculature of the retina and choroid in a noninvasive way using a technology and platform that is already integral and familiar to our offices. An OCT volume scan can now be taken and split into "slabs" that can then be viewed to assess the functional vasculature at different layers of the retina and choroid. Even though it is a very immature technology, already great advances are being made in our understanding of retinal diseases due to its ability to provide insights into parts of the retinal circulation that were previously poorly imaged. Furthermore, recent advances in imaging resolution, image quality, and software algorithms for interpretation of images are forwarding the technology as a whole. This textbook includes many authors who are experts in this new imaging modality from all over the world. It covers the technology in a comprehensive manner with most of the chapters focusing on retinal diseases and a few focusing on expanding indications of this technology in glaucoma, the anterior segment, uveitis, and oncology. We hope you will find this textbook a valuable addition to your library, providing a current state-of-the-art look at the technology!

David R. Chow, MD, FRCSC

Contributors

Francesco Bandello, MD, FEBO
Ophthalmologist
Department of Ophthalmology
University Vita-Salute
IRCCS Ospedale San Raffaele
Milan, Italy

Christophe Baudouin, MD, PhD
Professor and Chair of Ophthalmology
Quinze-Vingts National Ophthalmology Hospital &
Vision Institute
Paris, France

Rubens Belfort Jr., MD, PhD, MBA
Head Professor
Federal University of São Paulo (UNIFESP)
São Paulo, Brazil
President
Vision Institute
São Paulo, Brazil

Alan R. Berger, MDCM, FRCSC
Vitreoretinal Surgeon, St. Michael's Hospital
Vice Chairman, Clinical Services
Dept. of Ophthalmology and Vision Sciences
University of Toronto
Toronto, Canada

Adriano Carnevali, MD
Department of Ophthalmology
University Vita-Salute
IRCCS Ospedale San Raffaele
Milan, Italy
Department of Ophthalmology
University of "Magna Graecia"
Catanzaro, Italy

David R. Chow, MD, FRCSC
Assistant Professor
Department of Ophthalmology
St Michaels Hospital
University of Toronto
Fellowship Director and Co-Director
Toronto Retina Institute
Toronto, Ontario, Canada

Emily D. Cole, BS
New England Eye Center
Tufts University School of Medicine
Boston, Massachusetts

Federico Corvi, MD
Department of Ophthalmology
University Vita-Salute
IRCCS Ospedale San Raffaele
Milan, Italy

James G. Fujimoto, PhD
Elihu Thomson Professor of Electrical Engineering
Massachusetts Institute of Technology
Department of Electrical Engineering and Computer
Science and Research Lab of Electronics
Cambridge, Massachusetts

Alain Gaudric, MD
Emeritus Professor
Université Paris-Diderot, Sorbonne Paris-Cité
Hôpital Lariboisiere, AP-HP
Paris, France

Mostafa Hanout, MD, MSc
Clinical Fellow, Vitreoretinal Surgery
Department of Opthalmology and Visual Sciences
University of Toronto
St. Michael's Hospital
Toronto, Ontario, Canada

Stephanie Hayek, MD
Resident
Quinze-Vingts National Ophthalmology Hospital
Paris, France

Allen C. Ho, MD
Professor of Ophthalmology
Wills Eye Hospital Retina Service
Mid Atlantic Retina
Thomas Jefferson University
Philadelphia, Pennsylvania

Gábor Holló, MD, PhD, DSc
Professor of Ophthalmology
Head, Glaucoma and Perimetry Unit
Department of Ophthalmology, Semmelweis University,
Budapest
Budapest, Hungary

Nicholas A. Iafe, MD
Ophthalmology Resident
Stein Eye Institute
University of California Los Angeles
Los Angeles, California

Yasushi Ikuno, MD
Director and Founder
Ikuno Eye Center
Invited Professor
Graduate School of Medicine
Osaka University
Clinical Professor
Graduate School of Medical Sciences
Kanazawa University
Osaka, Japan

Peter K. Kaiser, MD
Chaney Family Endowed Chair in Ophthalmology
    Research
Professor of Ophthalmology
Cleveland, Ohio

Keyvan Koushan, MD, FRCSC
Vitreoretinal Surgeon
Mt. Sinai Hospital
University of Toronto
Toronto, Ontario, Canada

Valérie Krivosic, MD
Hôpital Lariboisiere, AP-HP
Service d'Opthalmologie
Reference Center for Rare Vascular Diseases of Brain
    and Eye (CERVCO)
Paris, France

Mark Lane, MD
Opthalmologist
University Hospitals Birmingham NHS Foundation Trust
Birmingham, United Kingdom

Ricardo Noguera Louzada, MD
Opthalmologist
Department of Ophthalmology
Federal University of Goiás
Goiânia, Brazil
New England Eye Center
Tufts University School of Medicine
Boston, Massachusetts

Adil El Maftouhi, OD
Centre Ophtalmologique Rabelais
Lyon, France

André Correa Maia de Carvalho, MD, PhD
Retina Clinic
São Paulo, Brazil
Department of Ophthalmology
Federal University of São Paulo (UNIFESP)
School of Medicine
São Paulo, Brazil

Colin A. McCannel, MD, FACS, FRCS
Associate Professor of Ophthalmology
Charles Drew University
Visiting Associate Professor
Stein Eye Institute
University of California, Los Angeles
Los Angeles, California

Tara A. McCannel, MD, PhD
Associate Clinical Professor of Ophthalmology
Director
Ophthalmic Oncology Center
Jules Stein Eye Institute
Los Angeles, CA, United States

Alexandra Miere, MD
Opthalmologist
Department of Ophthalmology
Centre Hospitalier Intercommunal de Créteil (CHIC)
Université Paris Est Créteil
Créteil, France

Meghna Motiani, MD
Resident Physician
Cedars Sinai Medical Center
Department of Internal Medicine
Los Angeles, California

Eric M. Moult, BSc
Massachusetts Institute of Technology
Department of Electrical Engineering and Computer
    Science and Research Lab of Electronics
Cambridge, Massachusetts

Eduardo A. Novais, MD
Retina Specialist and PhD Candidate
Department of Ophthalmology
Federal University of São Paulo (UNIFESP)
São Paulo, Brazil

Paulo Ricardo Chaves de Oliveira, MD
Ophthalmology degree
Faculdade de Ciências Médicas da Santa Casa de São Paulo
Retinal fellowship
Retina Clinic, São Paulo
Uveitis fellowship
Federal University of São Paulo (UNIFESP)
Retinal Research Fellow
Toronto Retina Institute, Canada
Retinal specialist
Instituto Panamericano da Visão
Goiânia, Brazil

Nopasak Phasukkijwatana, PhD, MD
International Fellow in Medical Retina
Stein Eye Institute, University of California Los Angeles
Los Angeles, California
Department of Ophthalmology
Faculty of Medicine Siriraj Hospital, Mahidol University
Bangkok, Thailand

Giuseppe Querques, MD, PhD
Head - Medical Retina & Imaging Unit
Department of Ophthalmology
University Vita Salute
IRCCS Ospedale San Raffaele
Milan, Italy

Lea Querques, MD
Ophthalmologist
Department of Ophthalmology
University Vita-Salute
IRCCS Ospedale San Raffaele
Milan, Italy

Carl D. Regillo, MD
Professor of Ophthalmology
Director of Wills Eye Hospital Retina Service
Mid Atlantic Retina
Thomas Jefferson University
Philadephia, Pennsylvania

André Romano, MD
Director
Neovista Eye Institute
São Paulo, Brazil
Adjunct Professor
University of Miami
Miller School of Medicine
Miami, Florida

Wasim A. Samara, MD
Postdoctoral Research Fellow
Wills Eye Hospital Retina Service
Mid Atlantic Retina
Thomas Jefferson University
Philadelphia, Pennsylvania
David Sarraf, MD
Clinical Professor of Ophthalmology
Stein Eye Institute
University of California Los Angeles
Los Angeles, California

Abtin Shahlaee, MD
Postdoctoral Research Fellow
Wills Eye Hospital Retina Service
Mid Atlantic Retina
Thomas Jefferson University
Philadelphia, Pennsylvania

Sumit Sharma, MD
Assistant Professor
Ophthalmology
Cleveland Clinic Cole Eye Institute
Cleveland, Ohio

Eric Souied, MD, PhD
Professor and Head
Department of Ophthalmology
Centre Hospitalier Intercommunal de Créteil (CHIC)
Université Paris Est Créteil
Créteil, France

Nadia K. Waheed, MD, MPH
Associate Professor of Ophthalmology
Tufts University School of Medicine
Director
Boston Image Reading Center
Tufts Medical Center/New England Eye Center
Boston Image Reading Center
New England Eye Center
Boston, Massachusetts

Taku Wakabayashi, MD
Ophthalmologist
Department of Ophthalmology
Osaka University Graduate School of Medicine
Osaka, Japan

1 Optical Coherence Tomography Angiography: Understanding the Basics

David R. Chow

Summary

Optical coherence tomography (OCT) angiography is an exciting new imaging modality that uses motion contrast to provide a noninvasive image of the retinal and choroidal vasculature. It is based on the acquisition of a three-dimensional (3D) volume OCT scan, which is then autosegmented and viewed en face to provide a view of the vasculature at any level of the retina or choroid. This chapter will review the basics of OCT angiography including the underlying technology, understanding the images obtained, and the evolving literature on these images in healthy eyes.

Keywords: optical coherence tomography angiography, fluorescein angiography, split spectrum amplitude decorrelation angiography, motion correction technology, autosegmentation

1.1 Introduction

Over the past 25 years, there has been a dramatic uptake in the usage of optical coherence tomography (OCT) as a noninvasive clinical tool to evaluate the structural anatomy of the macula and optic nerve head. Following its initial release as a research tool in the early 1990s, it reached mainstream clinical usage in the early 2000s with time domain technology, but really took off after 2005 with the release of Fourier domain or spectral domain OCT, which featured vast improvements in imaging resolution due to the higher scanning speeds coupled with motion correction technologies, such as eye tracking.[1] Present-day clinical retina practice is characterized by a combination of a clinical exam, OCT imaging to evaluate the structural anatomy of the macula, fluorescein angiography (FA) to evaluate the retinal vasculature and identify sites of leakage or staining, and on occasion indocyanine green (ICG) angiography to better evaluate the deeper choroidal circulation. Practice patterns as defined by the graduating Retina Fellows at the Retina Fellow Forum have shown an increasing reliance on OCT imaging to define clinical activity and a reducing usage of FA in the diagnosis and management of retinal diseases (▶ Fig. 1.1, ▶ Fig. 1.2). Since 1961 when FA was first used to image the retinal vasculature, it has been the gold standard for evaluating the retinal vasculature and retinal conditions characterized by leakage or staining. Although the capabilities of FA are well known to all retina specialists, so too are its risks, related to the intravenous injection of a dye, which is associated with nausea, vomiting, and anaphylactic shock.[2,3,4,5] It also requires a significant investment in time, equipment, and well-trained personnel to perform properly.

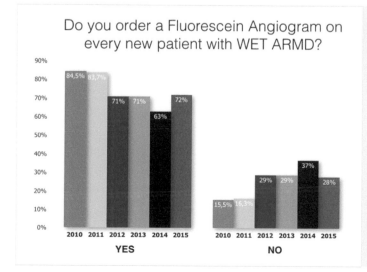

Fig. 1.1 Decreasing utilization of fluorescein angiography on new patients with WET ARMD. ARMD, age-related macular degeneration. (Data from graduating retina fellows at the North American Retina Fellow Forum, 2010–2015.)

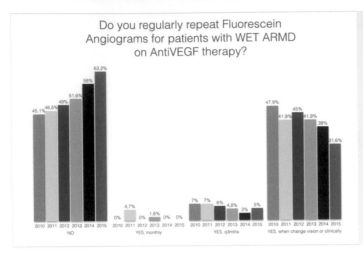

Fig. 1.2 Decreasing utilization of fluorescein angiography for patients with WET ARMD on Anti-VEGF therapy. ARMD, age-related macular degeneration; VEGF, vascular endothelial growth factor. (Data from graduating retina fellows at the North American Retina Fellow Forum, 2010-2015.)

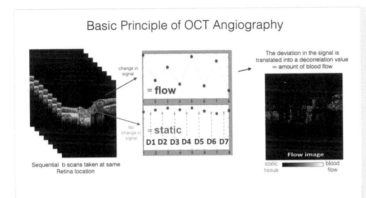

Fig. 1.3 Basic principle behind optical coherence tomography (OCT) angiography: sequential B-scans are taken of the retina at the exact same location. These scans are then compared to look for any changes in the signal. When present, this is deemed to represent movement in the retina at this location and inferred to represent blood flow. The deviation in the signal is mathematically assessed to provide a decorrelation signal representing the amount of blood flow at that point on the retina.

1.2 So What Is Optical Coherence Tomography Angiography and Why Is It So Exciting?

Over the last few years, the advances in imaging speeds and resolution of OCT platforms have resulted in the ability to detect blood flow by motion contrast and by extension provide an en face view of the retinal vasculature. The underlying principle behind this is that sequential B-scans are taken of the SAME retinal location and then subjected to analysis to determine if there was any change in the amplitude or phase of the scan. If changes are detected, this signifies movement in the retinal tissue of this location (▶ Fig. 1.3). The movement is inferred to be due to the flow of red blood cells in the vasculature, although there are occasional artifacts that can create a "false" impression of movement of the retina. The obtained signal can then be amplified (ex SSADA—split spectrum amplitude decorrelation angiography) and digitally processed to provide an en face view of the vasculature at different layers of the retina. Various motion correction technologies are also typically applied to the data to further enhance the quality (signal-to-noise ratio) of the obtained images (▶ Fig. 1.4).[6,7,8,9,10,11,12] The data are obtained in the typical manner that a structural OCT cube scan is done and in the same time sequence approximately 3 to 4 seconds. So, it importantly does not change the flow in a busy clinical retinal practice. Even better, and without question the most outstanding feature of OCT angiography (OCTA) is that this is all done without the injection of a contrast dye, so no intravenous (IV) and no risks of allergic reactions. OCTA is NONINVASIVE!

Motion correction technology

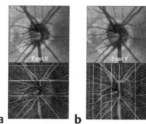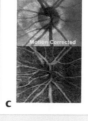

a   **b**   **c**

Fig. 1.4 Motion correction technology. **(a)** Horizontal priority fast transverse scans (Fast-X), **(b)** vertical priority fast transverse scans (Fast-Y) are taken, and then **(c)** software analyzed (Optovue's AngioVue system 2015) and merged to create a better-quality image free of motion artifacts including residual axial motion and transverse saccadic motions.

1.3 Making Sense of the Information Obtained in an OCTA

As every OCTA obtained is essentially a cube scan, it is a three-dimensional (3D) assessment of the retinal vasculature unlike traditional fluorescein or ICG angiography, which is two dimensional. As a result, to properly evaluate the data, an approach has to be taken to make sense of the volume of information. One approach could be to evaluate the scans from the inner retinal surface right down to the choroid in a continuous manner. This could be done manually or by creating a movie file of the scans. Both of these options require significant physician time and as a result there would be reluctance to use the data in this manner. In an attempt to simplify the data, most commercially available OCTA machines have taken the cube and split it into slabs to reflect a known anatomic layer

of the retinal vasculature, referred to as autosegmentation. For instance, the AngioVue software on the Optovue OCTA splits the volume cube up into the following four slabs:

1. Inner retinal slab extends from 3 µm below the internal limiting membrane to 15 µm below the inner plexiform layer. This incorporates the known anatomic location of the superficial retinal vascular plexus, which is generally what we see on traditional FA (▶ Fig. 1.5).

2. Middle retinal slab extends from 15 µm below the inner plexiform layer to 70 µm below the inner plexiform layer and incorporates the known location of the deep retinal capillary plexus. This plexus is poorly seen on traditional FA and beautifully seen on OCTA. Evaluating this region on OCTA is already providing insights into the pathology of conditions such as parafoveal telangiectasia (PFT) type 2b, paracentral acute middle maculopathy (PAMM), and retinal angiomatous proliferation (RAP), which we were unable to visualize clearly on traditional FA (▶ Fig. 1.6).

3. Outer retinal slab extends from 70 µm below the inner plexiform layer to 30 µm below the retinal pigment epithelium (RPE) reference line. This region anatomically corresponds to a part of the retina within which there is NEVER any vasculature in a normal individual. As a result, this slab should always be empty or blank unless there is pathology (▶ Fig. 1.7). This slab can be very useful to identify type 2 (subretinal) neovascular membranes.

4. Choriocapillaris extends from 30 µm below the RPE reference to 60 µm below the RPE reference. It incorporates the choriocapillaris and allows detection of early type 1 (sub-RPE) choroidal neovascular membranes (CNVM; ▶ Fig. 1.8).

Inner retinal slab
Extends from 3µm below ILM to 15µm below the inner plexiform layer

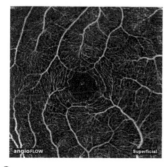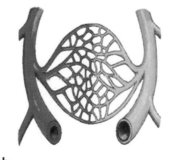

a   **b**

Fig. 1.5 Inner retinal slab (Optovue's AngioVue system) extends from 3 µ below the internal limiting membrane to 15 µ below the inner plexiform layer. **(a)** The optical coherence tomography (OCTA) image obtained looks very similar to the view obtained on traditional fluorescein angiography. **(b)** The traditional anatomic structure of the superficial retinal vascular plexus.

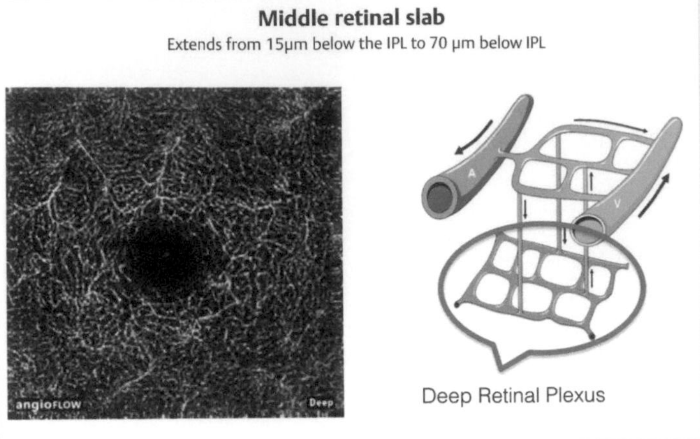

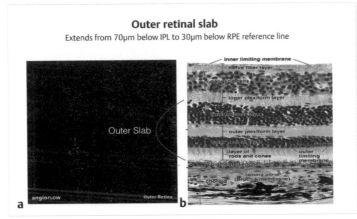

Fig. 1.6 Middle retinal slab (Optovue's AngioVue system) extends from 15 μm below the inner plexiform layer to 70 μm below the inner plexiform layer. **(a)** The optical coherence tomography (OCTA) image shows the deep retinal vascular plexus in detail never seen on traditional fluorescein angiography. This view of the deep retinal plexus is one of the more powerful new capabilities of OCTA. **(b)** The traditional view of the anatomy of the deep retinal plexus.

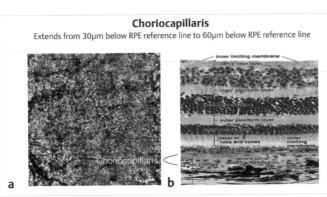

Fig. 1.7 Outer retinal slab (Optovue's AngioVue system) extends from 70 μm below the inner plexiform layer to 30 μm below the retinal pigment epithelium (RPE) reference line. **(a)** The optical coherence tomography (OCTA) image shows an empty box in normal individuals, as there is NEVER any vasculature in this part of a normal retina. **(b)** The anatomy of the slab imaged in the outer retinal slab.

Fig. 1.8 Choriocapillaris (Optovue's AngioVue system) extends from 30 μm below the retinal pigment epithelium (RPE) reference line to 60 μm below the RPE reference line. **(a)** The optical coherence tomography (OCTA) image shows speckled decorrelation signal representing the blood flow in the choriocapillaris. **(b)** The anatomy of the slab imaged is highlighted by the purple arch.

These four autosegmentation zones are then presented as four boxes on a single printout (▶ Fig. 1.9). In clinical practice, this view is easy to utilize and quite powerful at assessing the vasculature at each level of the retina and choriocapillaris. It should be noted that the autosegmentation zones sometimes fail to ideally present the pathology in a given zone particularly when the pathologic vessels do not fill or overfill the chosen segmentation slab. This is most evident in the choriocapillaris when visualizing CNVMs and needs to be appreciated particularly when trying to compare images of CNVM at successive visits where the response to therapy can be misinterpreted. We have found that for the evaluation of some CNVMs, manual manipulation of the boundaries of the slab

Standard OCTA report retina

Autosegmentation of 3D volume cube into 4 slabs
79 male with onset WET ARMD with type 1 CNVM in choriocapillaris

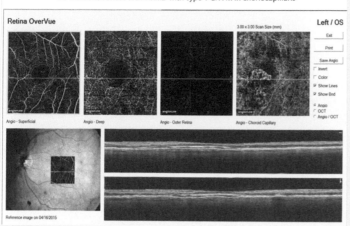

Fig. 1.9 Standard 3 × 3 mm optical coherence tomography (OCT) Angiogram Report of the Macula. Autosegmentation is applied to present the 3D cube data in four anatomic slabs: angio-superficial (superficial retinal capillary plexus), angio-deep (deep retinal capillary plexus), angio-outer retina, and angio-choroid capillary. The image presented is of a 79-year-old male with the onset of WET ARMD in the left eye. The OCT angiogram nicely illustrates a type 1 CNVM in the choriocapillaris slab. ARMD: age-related macular degeneration; CNVM: choroidal neovascular membrane.

Standard OCTA report optic nerve

Autosegmentation of 3D volume cube into four slabs
39 males with type 1 diabetes mellitus and onset PDR with NVD visible in vitreous slab

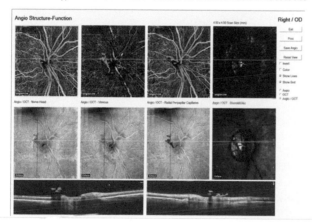

Fig. 1.10 Standard 3 × 3 mm optical coherence tomography (OCT) angiogram report of the optic nerve head. Autosegmentation is applied to present the 3D cube data in four anatomic slabs: angio-nerve head, angio-vitreous, angio-radial peripapillary capillaries, and angio-choroid disc. The image presented is of a 39-year-old male with type 1 diabetes mellitus who has developed NVD above the optic nerve head easily seen in the OCTA of the optic nerve on the vitreous slab. NVD, neovessels of the disc.

to be visualized is best to truly view the extent and nature of the CNVM complex.

Optic nerve head. In a manner similar to the scans obtained of the central macula, an OCTA can also be taken of the optic nerve head and peripapillary retina. These scans feature an autosegmentation option as well, which splits the view up into the following four zones (▶ Fig. 1.10):
1. The optic nerve head.
2. Above the optic nerve head or vitreous, which can be used to evaluate for the presence of neovessels of the disc or a vascularized hyaloid artery.
3. Radial peripapillary capillaries, which can be evaluated for ischemia and its potential role in

glaucoma. These capillaries are seen in exquisite detail on OCTA, while poorly viewed on traditional fluorescein and ICG angiography. This is a distinct advantage of OCTA over traditional imaging modalities.
4. Choroid/lamina cribrosa.

1.4 Nomenclature

Another important aspect to understand when evaluating OCTA images is that the intensity of the vessel, which you are visualizing on the printout, is a reflection of the amount of blood flow that was picked up with motion contrast or the decorrelation signal. There are, however, limitations on this as there is a minimal threshold or sensitivity limit, which reflects the time between the sequential B-scans that were taken. If the blood flow in a given region of the retina is SLOWER than the time between the B-scans chosen by a given manufacturer, then the OCTA will interpret that as absence of flow and no vasculature will be seen, even when there may be some. There is also a maximum threshold or saturation limit beyond which further flow is interpreted with the same signal. With traditional FA, we used the terms hyperfluorescence/hypofluorescence, leakage, staining, and blockage to reflect different types of pathology. Since fluorescein angiograms are dynamic with different phases, the pattern of fluorescence over time was a large part of the evaluation. OCTAs on the other hand are the same irrespective of time. That is, they are static, do not change, and will be the same whenever they are taken. We do NOT see leakage, staining, or blockage and as such will have to adjust our approach to interpreting some retinal diseases where we were engrained to look for dye leakage. Although the lack of leakage can be interpreted as a disadvantage for interpreting diseases such as central serous chorioretinopathy or CNVMs, it can also be an advantage, as the "true" anatomy of the pathologic vasculature will not get obscured over time.

1.5 Limitations of Optical Coherence Tomography Angiography

There are numerous current limitations of OCTA that need to be understood. The first is the sampling size. Initial OCTA were limited to 2 × 2 mm scans that allowed good visualization of only a very small central area of the macula, which was somewhat limiting. Current clinically released OCTA feature sample sizes of 3 × 3, 6 × 6, and 8 × 8 mm. There is hope that as technology improves we could eventually obtain scans of 12 × 12 mm, which are of high quality. At the present time at least it is highly recommended to use the 3 × 3 mm scans when looking for high-resolution images, as the pixel count in the 6 × 6 mm scans is the same as 3 × 3 mm, resulting in a significant reduction in image quality. We have found the 6 × 6 mm images are still useful, however, as a scanning angiogram to look for patterns of inner retinal ischemia such as is seen with retinal vein occlusions and severe diabetic disease. Another

limitation of OCTA is the artifact, which hinders obtaining usable images on many patients. Besides excessive movement, there are also surface artifacts and mirroring effects from the RPE that create confusing unreadable images. In a prospective study we conducted in our office, we found that in consecutive scans that 25.6% were deemed uninterpretable due to poor-quality images, mostly related to artifacts (unpublished data). This would seem like a large number of poor images, but it is important to remember that if the scan obtained is of poor quality, it can be repeated quickly and noninvasively. We have also found that the quality of images you obtain can be greatly improved through staff training.

1.6 Anatomic Discoveries in Normal Eyes with Optical Coherence Tomography Angiography

How does what we see on traditional FA compare to what is shown on an OCTA?

In a clever article by Spaide et al in 2015, simultaneous FA and OCTA on the same healthy patient were graded to determine what percentage of the vasculature seen on traditional FA was represented by the superficial versus the deep retinal vascular plexus as seen on the OCTA. They concluded that 95% of the vasculature seen on traditional FA represents the superficial retinal vascular plexus as seen on OCTA and that FA does a very poor job of imaging the deep retinal vascular plexus.[8]

1.6.1 Central versus Temporal Macula

Matsunaga et al in 2014 compared the vessel density in the inner and middle retina in healthy patients in the central, nasal, and temporal macula and found that the normal vessel density in both the inner and middle retina drops off significantly in the temporal macula compared to the central and nasal macula (temporal inner retina 22%, middle retina 28% vs. central macula inner retina 32%, middle retina 31% vs. nasal macula inner retina 31%, middle retina 31%).[13] Gadde et al in 2015 added that the vascular density appears to be greatest in the inferior sector around the foveal avascular zone (FAZ).[14]

1.6.2 Size of the foveal avascular zone

Samara et al in 2015 looked at 70 eyes of healthy patients and found that the size of the FAZ in the middle retina ($0.495 \pm 0.227\,mm^2$) was significantly larger than that of the inner retina ($0.266 \pm 0.097\,mm^2$) as assessed on OCTA. They found the size of the FAZ in both the inner and the middle retina was independent of age and sex but inversely correlated with central macular thickness and volume. The results obtained were consistent with previous measurements done with FA and adaptive optics.[15] Shahlaee et al recently published a similar study noting that the horizontal FAZ measurements of both the inner and the middle retina were larger than the vertical measurements and that there was considerably more variation in the size of the deep FAZ when interpreted by multiple graders.[16]

1.6.3 Radial Peripapillary Capillary Network

One of the distinct advantages of OCTA over FA is its ability to image the radial peripapillary capillary network, which is invisible on traditional FA. It has been long postulated that the reason why these vessels are NOT seen on FA is due to light scattering by the dense nerve fiber bundles located in this region.[8] Recent investigators have shown that ischemia of these capillaries may be used as a measure to monitor glaucoma patients.

1.6.4 Vascular Pattern of the Superficial versus Deep Retinal Plexus

Bonnin et al in 2015 reviewed the superficial retinal plexus (SRP) and deep retinal plexus (DRP) findings on OCTA in 41 consecutive normal eyes and suggested a novel anatomic pattern to the deep retinal capillary plexus. They agreed with others that the superficial retinal capillary plexus is arranged as a transverse capillary network forming an interconnected plexus between the feeding arterioles and draining venules and that there are vertically oriented interconnecting vessels to bridge the SRP and DRP. But uniquely, they suggested that the DRP is composed of polygonal units in which the capillaries converge radially toward a central capillary vortex, which then drains up into the superficial venules by the vertically oriented interconnecting venules.[17]

1.7 Conclusion

OCTA is an exciting new imaging modality that offers a number of advantages to clinical retina practice. It is a 3D imaging modality that provides high-quality static images of the retinal and choroidal vasculature without the need for any dye injections. The exams are quick and easy to obtain. The limitations of viewing artifacts, a small high-quality field of view, and lack of leakage will all be overcome as technology and our experience with it improve. Like all new technologies, academic validation is required and is currently ongoing. Already innumerable insights have been made using the technology to aid us in our ability to diagnose, manage, or understand retinal/choroidal disorders.

References

[1] Puliafito C. OCT angiography: the next era of OCTA technology emerges. Ophth Lasers Imaging Retina 2014;45:360

[2] López-Sáez MP, Ordoqui E, Tornero P, et al. Fluorescein-induced allergic reaction. Ann Allergy Asthma Immunol. 1998; 81(5):428–430

[3] Kwiterovich KA, Maguire MG, Murphy RP, et al. Frequency of adverse systemic reactions after fluorescein angiography. Results of a prospective study. Ophthalmology. 1991; 98(7). 1139–1142

[4] Ha SO, Kim DY, Sohn CH, Lim KS. Anaphylaxis caused by intravenous fluorescein: clinical characteristics and review of literature. Intern Emerg Med. 2014; 9(3):325–330

[5] Yannuzzi LA, Rohrer KT, Tindel LJ, et al. Fluorescein angiography complication survey. Ophthalmology. 1986; 93 (5):611–617

[6] Nagiel A, Sadda SR, Sarraf D. A promising future for optical coherence tomography angiography. JAMA Ophthalmol. 2015; 133(6):629–630

[7] Jia Y, Tan O, Tokayer J, et al. Split-spectrum amplitude-decorrelation angiography with optical coherence tomography. Opt Express. 2012; 20(4):4710–4725

[8] Spaide RF, Klancnik JM, Jr, Cooney MJ. Retinal vascular layers imaged by fluorescein angiography and optical coherence tomography angiography. JAMA Ophthalmol. 2015; 133(1): 45–50

[9] Zhang A, Zhang Q, Chen CL, Wang RK. Methods and algorithms for optical coherence tomography-based angiography: a review and comparison. J Biomed Opt. 2015; 20(10):100901

[10] Kraus MF, Potsaid B, Mayer MA, et al. Motion correction in optical coherence tomography volumes on a per A-scan basis using orthogonal scan patterns. Biomed Opt Express. 2012; 3 (6):1182–1199

[11] Schwartz DM, Fingler J, Kim DY, et al. Phase-variance optical coherence tomography. A technique for noninvasive angiography. Ophthalmology. 2014; 121(1):180–187

[12] Savastano MC, Lumbroso B. In vivo characterization of retinal vascularization morphology using optical coherence tomography angiography. Retina. 2015; 35(11):2196–203

[13] Matsunaga D, Yi J, Puliafito CA, Kashani AH. OCT angiography in healthy human subjects. Ophthalmic Surg Lasers Imaging Retina. 2014; 45(6):510–515

[14] Gadde SG, Anegondi N, Bhanushali D, et al. Quantification of vessel density in retinal optical coherence tomography angiography images using local fractal dimension. Invest Ophthalmol Vis Sci. 2016; 57(1):246–252

[15] Samara WA, Say EA, Khoo CT, et al. Correlation of foveal avascular zone size with foveal morphology in normal eyes using optical coherence tomography angiography. Retina. 2015; 35(11):2188–2195

[16] Shahlaee A, Pefkianaki M, Hsu J, Ho AC. Measurement of foveal avascular zone dimensions and its reliability in healthy eyes using optical coherence tomography angiography. American J Ophth. 2016; 161:50–55e.1

[17] Bonnin S, Mane V, Couturier A, et al. New insight into the macular deep vascular plexus imaged by optical coherence tomography angiography. Retina. 2015; 35:2347–2352

2 Optical Coherence Tomography Angiography Artifacts

Paulo Ricardo Chaves de Oliveira, Keyvan Koushan, André Maia, and David R. Chow

Summary

Optical coherence tomography angiography (OCTA) is a new technology that allows the dye-free study of the chorioretinal vasculature. Many efforts are under way to better understand how it could be effectively incorporated into our clinical practice and enhance the care of our patients. However, as with every imaging modality, artifacts can degrade the quality of images in OCTA. Recognizing these artifacts is essential in order to avoid misinterpretations and erroneous diagnosis. In this chapter, we review some of the most common OCTA artifacts, including segmentation errors, motion-related artifacts, vessel projection, and shadowing effects.

Keywords: artifacts, motion artifact, optical coherence tomography angiography, projection artifact, shadowing effect

2.1 Introduction

First introduced in 1991, by Huang et al, optical coherence tomography (OCT)[1] is an integral part of the workup of every retina patient. The qualitative and quantitative assessment of the retina through OCT has revolutionized the field of opthalmology. OCT has helped ophthalmologists with their diagnostic and treatment decisions for many years. However, as in every imaging system, the resulting image is subject to artifacts and "information" may be inadvertently acquired, subtracted, or added to the image originally captured. That could be related, but not limited to, inappropriate operator technique, patient limitations (e.g., motion during exam), or software "failure."[2] As a result, when assessing regular cross-sectional OCT images, segmentation errors, degraded images, off-center images, and other alterations have been reported.[2,3]

Optical coherence tomography angiography (OCTA) is a novel technology based on principles of OCT, and therefore, is also prone to artifacts. Recognizing their presence is important to avoid misinterpretations and to improve exam accuracy. This could be achieved by understanding how the technology works to produce a comprehensive analysis of structural OCT (conventional B-scan), en face OCT, and OCTA. Considering that OCTA technology is still at its beginning stages, there are only a limited number of reports (e.g., works by Spaide et al[4] and Chen et al[5]) on the issue of OCTA artifacts. Our goal in this chapter is to help the reader gain a better understanding of the artifacts that are commonly encountered in OCTA images.

2.2 How does Optical Coherence Tomography Angiography work?

Briefly, as it has already been described in a previous chapter, OCTA can detect flow by measuring the changes (decorrelation) in the reflected OCT signal intensity (amplitude) between consecutive cross-sectional B-scans taken at the exact same position or by assessing changes in the phase of the reflected light waves over time (phase variance). A combination of both is also possible.[2,4,6,7] In general terms, the commercially available machines incorporate different algorithms to assess the alterations in the OCT signal of successive B-scans taken at the same place. In any case, static tissue will show little change, while moving objects—such as red blood cells—will have significant variations. Those variations are assumed to originate from flow. As a result, blood motion contrast is generated and AngioFlow maps are created.[4]

2.3 Motion Artifacts

Since OCTA detects erythrocyte movement to generate contrast, it is extremely motion sensitive and prone to motion artifacts.[6] Movements that cause artifacts can occur in the axial direction (from heartbeat and respiration) or in the transverse direction (as in saccadic movements of the eye). As a result, the acquired volume might not accurately correspond to the real retinal architecture.[8] Algorithms, such as the split-spectrum amplitude-decorrelation angiography (SSADA), lower the resolution of axial OCT in order to minimize sensitivity to axial movement.[4] One advantage of this approach is that it does not affect the analysis of OCTA images, since most of the flow signal in the ocular fundus is in the transverse rather than axial dimension.[9] However, transverse movements are still a major problem. These movements are recognized as white lines in the OCTA en face scans. Some systems use software-based motion correction by creating two orthogonal volumes from a Fast-X (fast B-scans acquired in horizontal direction) and a Fast-Y (fast B-scans acquired in vertical direction) raster scans. The two orthogonal volumes are then merged to obtain a single volume with better signal quality.[8] Summarily, the

software tries to estimate and correct the eye motion for each A-scan in the two volumes (▶ Fig. 2.1). Unfortunately, while correcting small saccades and fixation losses, the system can introduce artifacts of its own, such as double vessels, stretching, and crisscrossing defects (▶ Fig. 2.2).[4,8] In addition, gross eye movements cannot be compensated and might result in poor-quality images (▶ Fig. 2.3). In a recent analysis of image quality when using the RTVue XR Avanti with AngioVue software (Optovue, Fremont, CA), we found that

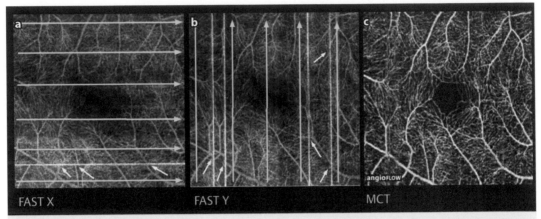

Fig. 2.1 Motion correction technology incorporated to the Optovue XR Avanti with AngioVue software. **(a)** Fast-X and **(b)** Fast-Y raster scan. Note the white lines (yellow arrows) due to motion artifacts, before the incorporation of motion correction technology. **(c)** The two orthogonal volumes are then merged to form a single optical coherence tomography angiography volume. MCT, motion corrected volume.

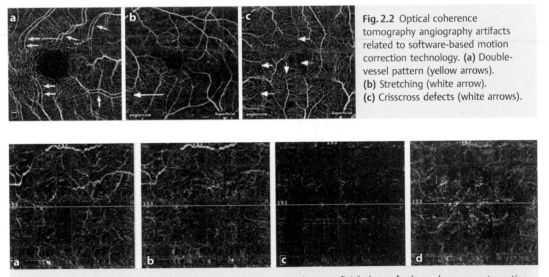

Fig. 2.2 Optical coherence tomography angiography artifacts related to software-based motion correction technology. **(a)** Double-vessel pattern (yellow arrows). **(b)** Stretching (white arrow). **(c)** Crisscross defects (white arrows).

Fig. 2.3 Poor-quality optical coherence tomography angiograms (**a**, superficial plexus; **b**, deep plexus; **c**, outer retina; **d**, choriocapillaris) due to gross eye movements. Neither quantitative nor qualitative assessment would be possible in this situation.

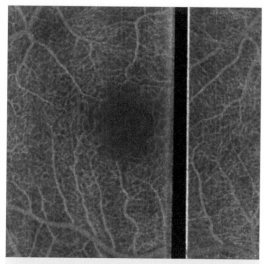

Fig. 2.4 Blinking artifact. Note the black line in the optical coherence tomography angiography image. Another capture protocol should be done by the operator.

motion artifacts counted for the majority of poor-quality exams (i.e., those scans for which neither qualitative nor quantitative assessment could be made) and was significantly higher in patients with a vision acuity of worse than 20/70, probably due to their difficulty in maintaining fixation during the acquisition process (PRC, Oliveira, MD; DR, Chow, MD, FRCS; 2016). Faster scanning speeds and eye-tracking technology might help improve these issues.

Blinking is another source of artifacts while obtaining images and appears as black lines on OCT angiograms (▶ Fig. 2.4). The OCT signal is blocked from getting to the retina and no flow is detected.

2.4 Projection Artifacts

This is probably the most common artifact and is virtually present in every OCTA exam. It corresponds to the fluctuation of light that passes through moving blood in the inner retinal vessels and is projected back to the deeper reflective layers such as the retinal pigment epithelium (RPE). Since that light also changes over time, those deeper layers will seem to have blood vessels with the pattern of the overlying retinal vessels (▶ Fig. 2.5).[4,5,10,11] Projection artifacts can especially cause falsely positive results during identification and quantification of choroidal neovascular (CNV) membranes. Some OCTA systems include the option of eliminating the projection artifacts. But in so doing, they can produce artificially low signal intensity in areas of pathologic vessels, leading to underestimation of the real magnitude of the lesions. When this secondary artifact happens, the projection artifact is actually substituted by a shadow artifact, leaving gaps in the neovascular network. Zhang et al published a "projection-resolved" algorithm, which improves the quality of the resulting OCTA after the suppression of the projection artifact. But, as stated by the authors, this system remains imperfect, leaving minor gaps in the deep retinal plexus and residual projection artifact in the RPE layer.[10] As the OCTA technology continues to improve, it will be a matter of time before issues related to projection artifacts are resolved.

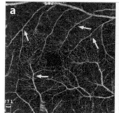
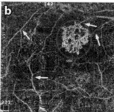
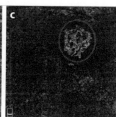

Fig. 2.5 optical coherence tomography angiography angiomaps in a case of a type 2 choroidal neovascular membrane (CNVM). Presence and suppression of projection artifacts: **(a)** the superficial retinal vessels are projected onto deeper layers and are visible at the level of the outer retina **(b;** yellow arrows), also overlapping the neovascular complex (blue dashed line). **(c)** Suppression of the projection artifact. The superficial vessels are no longer visible. However, shadows and gaps (red asterisks) are left and may compromise the quantitative assessment of the neovascular network.

2.5 Shadowing / Masking Effect

In order to reduce false-flow images generated by fluctuations of noise, OCTA is set to only process images from a minimum signal threshold. Thereby, areas of low signal will generate no flow when comparing one image to another.[4] This gives rise to another type of artifact related to a shadowing or masking effect. Signal attenuation may occur due to optically dense materials, such as cataracts, hemorrhages, and RPE.[4,12] More anterior media opacities will likely attenuate the OCTA signal all the way from the inner to the outer retinal layers. However, more posterior optically dense structures, such as pigment epithelium detachments (PED), will cause low signal intensity just posterior to that specific structure. Those low-signal regions (diffuse or locally distributed) will seem to have no flow, creating a false-negative OCTA flow pattern (▶ Fig. 2.6, ▶ Fig. 2.7).[4,5] That may explain why the choriocapillaris vessels, with a low signal under the intact RPE, are difficult to display using OCTA. In areas of RPE atrophy, however, the deeper choroidal vessels may become apparent (▶ Fig. 2.8). Another common manifestation of this shadowing artifact is masking of CNV complexes when they are located under PEDs in neovascular age-related macular degeneration.

2.6 Segmentation Artifact

The software in all OCTA systems incorporates algorithms to automatically segment the retina into en face slabs. The algorithms involved in the generation of these slabs are created assuming a healthy retina. Therefore, when imaging pathology, segmentation artifacts due to inaccurate estimation of en face slabs are possible. When this type of error happens, the AngioFlow images may not accurately reflect the vascular distribution that is expected for different retinal layers (▶ Fig. 2.9).[4] In such cases, concomitant OCT B-scan analysis and manual adjustment of the slab boundaries can help achieve more accurate exam interpretation.

2.7 Other Considerations

Since OCTA can only detect flow above a minimum threshold, sectors of slower flow than the slowest detectable flow will not show changes between consecutive B-scans and are displayed as dark areas (false-negative flow pattern). This could be one of the reasons why microaneurysms are not always detected by this technique.[4,6] On the other hand, OCTA systems are configured to display small decorrelation values, as observed in slow detectable flows, as bright pixels. Increasing the

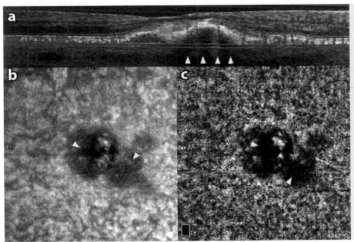

Fig. 2.6 False-negative optical coherence tomography angiography (OCTA) flow pattern caused by shadowing effect. **(a)** Cross-sectional OCT scan showing hyporeflective areas under the pigment epithelium detachment (PED) due to shadowing effect (yellow arrowheads). Blue lines correspond to the boundaries of choriocapillaris slab; corresponding 3 × 3 mm **(b)** OCT en face and **(c)** OCTA image at the level of choriocapillaris slab showing false low-flow areas (yellow arrowheads) due to shadowing effect and low OCT signal.

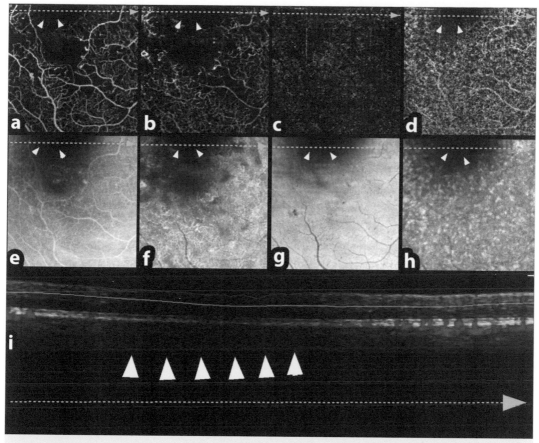

Fig. 2.7 Media opacity and shadowing effect on optical coherence tomography (OCT) angiography of a 50-year-old patient, with proliferative diabetic retinopathy and posterior subcapsular cataract in his right eye. A dark area is observed in all OCT angiography slabs (**a**, superficial vascular plexus; **b**, deep vascular plexus; **c**, outer retina; **d**, choriocapillaris; yellow arrowheads) that could correspond to a nonperfused area. However, that is a shadowing effect (loss of OCT signal) caused by an anterior media opacity (cataract). Note the corresponding hyporeflective on en face OCT (**e–h**; yellow arrowheads) and cross-sectional OCT (**i**; yellow arrowheads). Green dashed lines indicate the position of the OCT B-scan shown in (**i**).

flow speed will only increase the brightness of the displayed vessels until a certain limit, when the system is said to saturate. From this point, additional increase in the flow velocity will not lead to additional increase of the vascular brightness. As a result, quantitative assessment of flow speed using OCTA technology is currently unreliable, although it is likely to be possible in the near future (see Chapter 18).[4]

OCTA is a new exciting technology that has a promising future. The possibility of evaluating different retinal vascular layers in a noninvasive manner has been enhancing our understanding of different retinal vascular diseases. However, as described in this chapter, this technology is not free of artifacts. Understanding these artifacts is crucial for the proper utilization of this technology in clinical practice. Recognition of these artifacts is also important for the development of OCTA-based clinical trials and for establishing common terminology used in reading centers. In the near future, faster scanning speeds and software improvements are expected to reduce the frequency and magnitude of these artifacts.

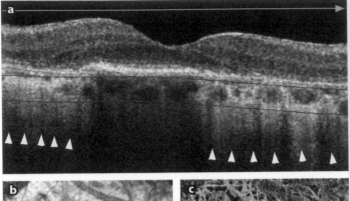

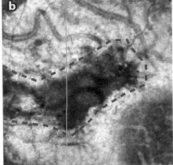

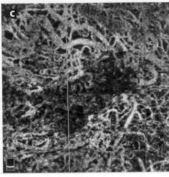

Fig. 2.8 An 82-year-old female patient with dry age-related macular degeneration and geographic atrophy in her right eye. **(a)** Cross-sectional optical coherence tomography (OCT) showing areas of choroidal hyper-reflectivity under the retinal pigment epithelial (RPE) and choriocapillaris atrophy due to increased light transmission (yellow arrowheads). **(b)** En face OCT showing hyper-reflectivity in areas of RPE atrophy (outside blue dashed line). The green line indicates the position of OCT cross-section shown in **(a)**. **(c)** Choroidal vessels are visible on the OCTA flow map under the RPE atrophy (outside blue dashed line). Areas where the RPE is present (inside blue dashed line), the deeper choroidal vessels are not visible due to OCT signal attenuation. The green line indicates the position of OCT cross-section shown in **(a)**.

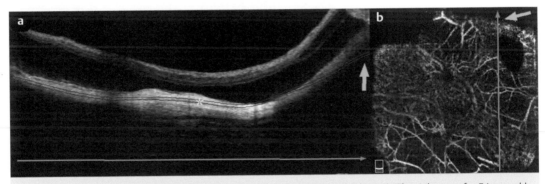

Fig. 2.9 Segmentation artifact in optical coherence tomography angiography (OCTA). The right eye of a 54-year-old high myopic patient. The different shape of this pathologic eye leads to autosegmentation errors. The choriocapillaris was initially selected. However, the slab boundaries shown in the structural OCT are crossing different layers (a, red lines), including the sclera (yellow asterisk). A portion "leaving" the eye is also demonstrated (a, green arrow) and is displayed as dark area in the **(b)** AngioFlow map. The majority of vessels shown in the OCTA flow image are projections of the superficial vessels. The blue line indicates the position of OCT cross-section shown in **(a)**.

References

[1] Huang D, Swanson EA, Lin CP, et al. Optical coherence tomography. Science. 1991; 254(5035):1178–1181

[2] Chhablani J, Krishnan T, Sethi V, Kozak I. Artifacts in optical coherence tomography. Saudi J Ophthalmol. 2014; 28(2): 81–87

[3] Han IC, Jaffe GJ. Evaluation of artifacts associated with macular spectral-domain optical coherence tomography. Ophthalmology. 2010; 117(6):1177–1189.e4

[4] Spaide RF, Fujimoto JG, Waheed NK. Image artifacts in optical coherence tomography angiography. Retina. 2015; 35(11): 2163–2180

[5] Chen FK, Viljoen RD, Bukowska DM. Classification of image artefacts in optical coherence tomography angiography of the choroid in macular diseases. Clin Experiment Ophthalmol. 2016; 44(5):388–399

[6] de Carlo TE, Romano A, Waheed NK, Duker JS. A review of optical coherence tomography angiography (OCTA). Int J Retina Vitreous. 2015; 1(1):5

[7] Palejwala NV, Jia Y, Gao SS, et al. Detection of nonexudative choroidal neovascularization in age-related macular degeneration with optical coherence tomography angiography. Retina. 2015; 35(11):2204–2211

[8] Kraus MF, Potsaid B, Mayer MA, et al. Motion correction in optical coherence tomography volumes on a per A-scan basis using orthogonal scan patterns. Biomed Opt Express. 2012; 3 (6):1182–1199

[9] Jia Y, Tan O, Tokayer J, et al. Split-spectrum amplitude-decorrelation angiography with optical coherence tomography. Opt Express. 2012; 20(4):4710–4725

[10] Zhang M, Hwang TS, Campbell JP, et al. Projection-resolved optical coherence tomographic angiography. Biomed Opt Express. 2016; 7(3):816–828

[11] Zhang A, Zhang Q, Wang RK. Minimizing projection artifacts for accurate presentation of choroidal neovascularization in OCT micro-angiography. Biomed Opt Express. 2015; 6(10): 4130–4143

[12] de Carlo TE, Baumal CR. Advances in optical coherence tomography angiography. US Ophthalmic Rev. 2016; 9(1):37–40

3 Current Optical Coherence Tomography Angiography Clinical Systems

Sumit Sharma and Peter K. Kaiser

Summary

Currently four optical coherence tomography angiography (OCTA) devices are commercially available on the market, and there are other companies working to produce their own device. Each of these devices are based on different systems and use different techniques to generate the angiographic images. In this chapter, we will review the methods used and the differences between the devices.

Keywords: optical coherence tomography angiography, OCTA, commercial devices, optovue Angio-Vue, zeiss AngioPlex, topcon DRI Triton, nidek AngioScan

3.1 Introduction

Currently, there are four commercially available systems that perform optical coherence tomography angiography (OCTA): Zeiss AngioPlex (Carl Zeiss Meditec, Dublin, CA), Optovue Angioview (Optovue, Inc., Fremont, CA), Nidek AngioScan (Nidek Company Ltd, Gamagori, Japan), and the Topcon DRI OCT Triton (Topcon Corporation, Tokyo, Japan). Other commercially available spectral domain devices are working on developing systems and there are non–Food and Drug Administration (FDA)-approved swept-source devices in clinical development. The AngioPlex, AngioView, and AngioScan systems are based on spectral domain OCT (SDOCT) systems, while the DRI OCT is based on a swept-source OCT system (SSOCT). All systems utilize different processing algorithms to transform the OCT B-scan images into an angiographic image. We will review the methods used and the differences between the devices in this chapter. As this is a rapidly developing field, many of the techniques and differences highlighted in this chapter may change in the very near future, and better systems are likely shortly.

3.2 Optovue AngioVue

The underlying technology of the Optovue Angio-Vue system is the Avanti SDOCT wide-field imaging system. The Avanti system utilizes an 840-nm light source with a bandwidth of 50 nm and has an A-scan rate of 70,000 scans per second.[1] The system has an axial resolution of 5 μm, transverse resolution of 15 μm, and an A-scan depth of approximately 3 mm. The fast scanning speed is needed for acquiring the large angiography dataset in a reasonable time.

To generate the OCTA image, the system acquires three-dimensional (3D) data acquisition volumes consisting of 304 × 304 A-scans in approximately 3 seconds and then uses orthogonal registration and merging of two consecutive scan volumes to obtain the 3 × 3, 6 × 6, or 8 × 8 mm OCTA volumes. AngioVue DualTrac Motion Correction Technology (MCT) provides enhanced flow visualization and ultraprecise-motion correction. During the OCTA capture, infrared (IR) video is used for tracking on each fast-X and fast-Y scans so that each OCTA image will have minimum eye motion artifacts. The tracking improves patient comfort by allowing blinks and fixation drifts during acquisition.

Before motion correction, the system utilizes a split-spectrum amplitude-decorrelation angiography (SSADA) algorithm to extract the OCTA information[2] from each fast-X and fast-Y OCTA scan. The SSADA algorithm detects motion in the blood vessels by measuring the variation in the reflected OCT signal amplitude between consecutive scans.[1,3] The decorrelation (1-correlation) of the signal amplitude between consecutive B-scans is then calculated allowing for evaluation of the contrast between tissue with motion and that without motion, that is, blood flow. Since decorrelation can also be generated by bulk eye motion, the SSADA algorithm splits the original full spectrum to 11 subspectrum OCTA images. While this lowers the resolution of the image, it also results in less susceptibility to eye motion and a wider coherence gate over which a moving blood cell can interfere with adjacent structures. Each of the split-spectrum images contains a different speckle pattern that also has independent information on flow. By combining the images from the various spectral bands, the flow signal is intensified. Increasing the number of spectral bands that are analyzed enhances the signal-to-noise ratio and increases the ability to detect flow.

The use of the orthogonal OCTA volumes is necessary to apply motion correction algorithms. The postprocessing MCT increases the number of patients that can be successfully scanned compared to independent use of real-time tracking and enhances microvascular flow visualization. MCT is necessary to minimize OCTA artifacts related to microsaccades and fixation changes.[4] Without motion correction, bright lines would appear in the OCTA image due to saccade motion. Since an eye takes 1 millisecond to move 300 μm, an OCT device would need to have 10 kHz tracking speed to get 30-μm accuracy. While 1-kHz laser tracking systems could perform this tracking, it would be very expensive. Most scanners use image tracking that tracks at a 15- to 30-Hz speed—in general too slow for OCTA. The AngioVue system uses a sophisticated algorithm that performs a rough axial correction in the first stage, then a full optimization in the second stage to produce the merged image. The motion-corrected data improves signal-to-noise ratio and corrects for z-motion artifacts. This requires considerable computational power. The registered and merged data output is used to apply the angiography algorithm.

The flow information is then presented as an en face image with segmentation utilized to show different levels of vasculature. The AngioVue software generates four default en face imaging zones: the superficial plexus, the deep plexus, the outer retina, and the choriocapillaris.[5] The software can also be manipulated to show a custom region of interest.

The AngioVue software also does quantitative analysis of the OCT angiograms. The new quantification tool is called AngioAnalytics. This tool provides numerical data about flow and nonflow areas. This information is used to generate a flow density map that may be used to track the change in perfusion density over time. This data should be taken with a grain of salt, however, as the SSADA algorithm is felt to saturate at higher velocities such as those seen in larger vessels.[6] The software also allows the user to draw the borders of the choroidal neovascularization and the software will calculate the drawn area and the vessel area. It also generates maps of nonflow areas that can be tracked over time. Most of the new software is still in its infancy and each iteration adds more features.

3.3 Carl Zeiss Meditec AngioPlex

The Carl Zeiss Meditec AngioPlex system is based on an upgraded Cirrus 5000 instrument. This SDOCT system has an A-scan rate of 68,000 A-scans per second with a light source centered on 840 nm with a bandwidth of 90 nm. The system has an axial resolution of 5 μm, transverse resolution of 15 μm, and an A-scan depth of 2.0 mm. The system incorporates a retinal tracking technology to track and compensate for eye movements in real time, and using a proprietary algorithm allows the device to rescan areas that may have been affected by motion. This system also allows for registration between visits so that the exact same area can be imaged on consecutive visits. Postacquisition motion correction software is not part of the device.

There are three patterns available for imaging on the AngioPlex: 3 × 3, 6 × 6, and 8 × 8 mm. The OCTA analysis shows six en face slabs representing the inner capillary plexus, outer capillary plexus, the outer retina, which should normally be avascular, the choriocapillaris, the choroid, and vasculature above the vitreoretinal interface, which should also normally be avascular. The AngioPlex software also combines three of the retinal en face slabs to provide visualization of microvasculature in the entire retina and also uses color mapping to show flow in the superficial, deep, and avascular layers as red, green, and blue, respectively, in a color depth–encoded slab. As with AngioVue, the AngioPlex device also captures consecutive B-scans; the differences lie in how the data is then processed by the device to generate the final en face images. The AngioPlex device uses the optical microangiography (OMAG) algorithm to generate the final en face OCTA images instead of the SSADA algorithm.[7]

The OMAG algorithm examines the signal differences in successive B-scans at the same location and records these as vectors utilizing both the amplitude and the phase of the signal, which are then used to create a picture of changes in the microscopic structures encountered.[8,9] The resulting image relies on the contrast in the OCT signal created by motion of scattering elements, which is primarily expected to be due to flow of erythrocytes through vessels. OMAG allows for high-sensitivity imaging of capillary flow. The high sensitivity of OMAG makes it susceptible to bulk-motion artifacts and the algorithm can only be utilized with precise-motion correction.[3,10] Because the bulk-motion correction and precise-motion correction are part of the implementation in AngioPlex, the device can offer high sensitivity to microvascular flow, with no loss of axial resolution that occurs with use of narrower spectrum of wavelength.

3.4 Nidek RS-3000 Advance Optical Coherence Tomography

The Nidek RS-3000 Advance OCT is a SDOCT system with AngioScan OCTA software. Like the Cirrus AngioPlex, OCTA can be added to recent OCT devices via a software update. In some cases, a replacement of the PC unit is required. The AngioScan software uses the tracing high-definition (HD) function of the RS-3000 to track eye movements, which is necessary for the OCTA software to insure the sequential images are taken from the same place. The scan size ranges from 3 mm to a maximum of 9 mm. Using a composite function, a wide-angle panoramic OCT image up to $12 \times 9 \, mm^2$ is also possible. The resulting image can be imaged en face and with false color representing the depths of the vascular channels. The software can remove the projection artifacts from the inner vasculature when viewing the outer vasculature.

Proprietary software offers measurement of areas of ischemia, area of the foveal avascular zone, and a density map of the vasculature. A unique mode of the AngioScan software displays choroidal neovascular membrane (CNV) blood flow independent of the normal vasculature. This makes it easier to highlight areas of neovascularization. Like the other devices, this software is still in its infancy and is undergoing significant improvement as software algorithms get optimized.

3.5 Topcon DRI OCT Triton

The Topcon DRI OCT Triton is an SSOCT system that has a number of advantages over SDOCT systems. The DRI OCT uses a 1,050-nm light source with a 100,000 A-scan per second scan rate.[11] Since the system uses a longer wavelength light source compared to SDOCT devices, it has improved penetration into tissue; therefore, it should theoretically be able to image the choroid better. Additionally, the use of a 1050-nm light source should be more comfortable for the patient given it is in the IR spectrum and is not visible to the patient. Similar to the other two devices described earlier, the DRI OCT can generate en face OCTA images of either 3×3 or 6×6 mm. The DRI OCT includes motion correction to help account for patient movement.

The DRI OCT uses yet another proprietary algorithm to produce the OCTA images—OCTA ratio analysis (OCTARA).[12] The Topcon OCTARA algorithm does not require splitting the spectrum and

thus maintains the full axial resolution. Unlike the other two devices described earlier, the faster speed of the SSOCT system allows for each B-scan position to be scanned four times. The B-scans at each location are then registered to each other and the OCTA images are generated by computing a ratio-based result between corresponding image pixels. This represents a relative measurement of OCT signal amplitude change while optimizing angiographic visualization over the retina and choroid. The system suppresses motion artifacts by averaging multiple registered B-scans.

The DRI OCT software displays en face OCTA images corresponding to the superficial and deep capillary plexus as well as the choriocapillaris by default. In addition, the corresponding OCT cross-sectional image, IR fundus image, and en face OCT are also shown for comparison.

3.6 Others

There are a few other companies currently developing OCTA systems, but they were not readily commercially available at the time of completion of this chapter. These include the Spectralis OCTA (Heidelberg Engineering, Inc., Heidelberg, Germany) and the Canon Angio eXpert (Canon, Inc., Tokyo, Japan). Each of these devices uses a different software and hardware approach. Information on the specifics of each device was not available at the time of publication of this chapter.

3.7 Comparisons

Unfortunately, there have been no published studies comparing the en face OCTA images generated by the various commercially available systems to each other in the same patient. As a point of reference, example images from some of these systems in normal patients are shown in ▶ Fig. 3.1, ▶ Fig. 3.2, and ▶ Fig. 3.3. ▶ Fig. 3.4 and ▶ Fig. 3.5 show examples of CNV on the AngioView and AngioPlex. ▶ Fig. 3.6 shows an image of geographic atrophy assessed by the OMAG algorithm, in the Zeiss AngioPlex software.

A comparison was made between the AngioVue and the AngioPlex systems. The AngioPlex system was found to have a shorter acquisition time and fewer motion artifacts compared to the AngioVue system for both patients and healthy controls.[13] This was felt to be related to the fact that the AngioPlex systems uses active eye tracking algorithms. The use of active eye tracking allowed the

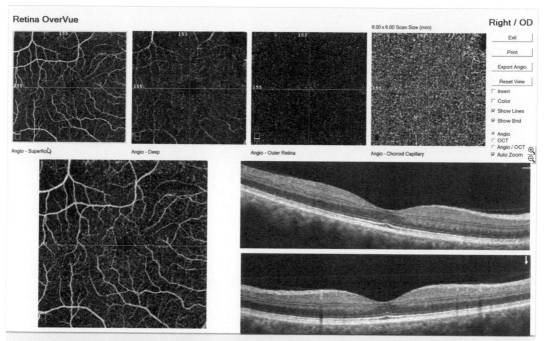

Fig. 3.1 Normal patient imaged and analyzed on Optovue AngioVue software. The software shows four optical coherence tomography (OCT) angiographic views: superficial capillary plexus, deep capillary plexus, the outer retina, and the choriocapillaris as well the corresponding horizontal and vertical OCT B-scans. The red and green lines on the B-scans correlate to the area being analyzed by the OCTA algorithm in the large OCTA image displayed. These can be manually manipulated in the software to show a targeted area of interest.

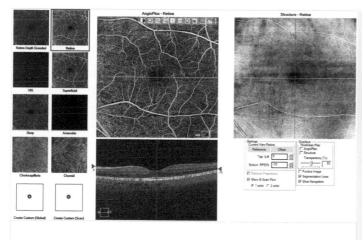

Fig. 3.2 Normal patient imaged and analyzed on the Zeiss AngioPlex software. The software shows eight optical coherence tomography (OCT) angiographic views: a composite false color full OCTA image, a composite full OCTA image without false color, the vitreoretinal interface, superficial capillary plexus, deep capillary plexus, the outer retina, the choriocapillaris, and the choroid as well as the corresponding horizontal OCT B-scan image. The area of the retina being imaged is indicated on the B-scan as the area between the two purple lines. These can be manually manipulated in the software to show a targeted area of interest. The red areas overlaid on the B-scan correspond to area of flow as detected by the algorithm.

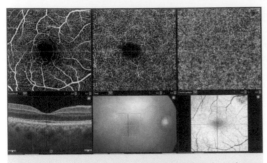

Fig. 3.3 Normal patient imaged and analyzed on the Topcon DRI Triton software. The software shows three angiographic views: superficial capillary plexus, deep capillary plexus, and the choriocapillaris as well as the corresponding horizontal optical coherence tomography (OCT) B-scan, a red free fundus image, and the en face OCT scan. The green lines on the B-scan correlate to the area being analyzed by the OCTA algorithm.

system to account for both microsaccades and voluntary eye movements. No mention was made of the difference in the ability to detect pathology on either system.

3.8 Conclusion

The field of OCTA is rapidly developing with multiple new devices that will soon be commercially available. Each of these devices utilizes a different setup and uses different algorithms to generate the en face OCTA images. One must be acutely aware of the differences between the devices and the types of artifacts that are generated by OCTA in order to accurately analyze the images. There is still much work that must be done to determine which of these algorithms and approaches provides the best OCTA images with the fewest artifacts.

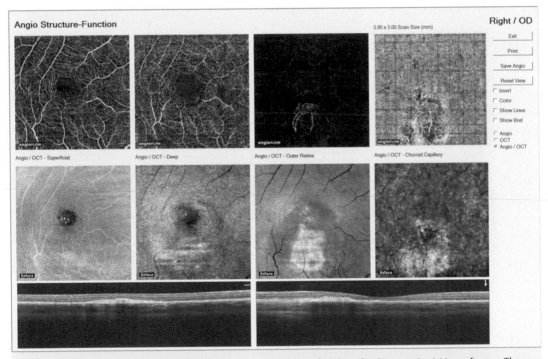

Fig. 3.4 Choroidal neovascular membrane (CNV) as imaged and analyzed on the Optovue AngioVue software. The superficial and deep capillary plexus images are fairly normal; however, the outer retina and choriocapillaris images show a branching vascular network corresponding to a CNV.

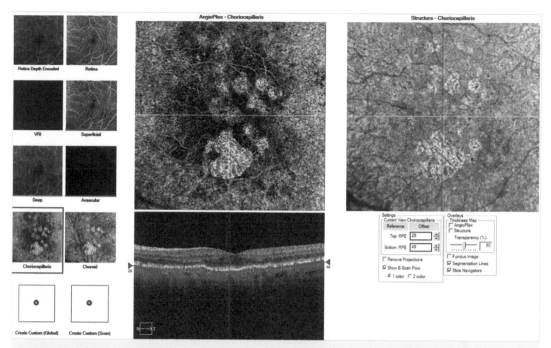

Fig. 3.5 CNV imaged and analyzed on the Zeiss AngioPlex software. The choriocapillaris and choroid images show a branching vascular network corresponding to a CNV. Of note, the images and detail available are different from the images obtained on the Optovue device, but these are from different patients.

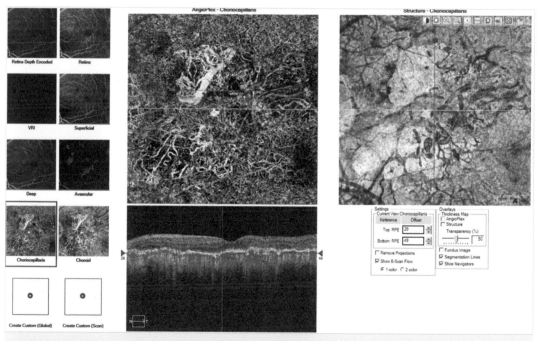

Fig. 3.6 Geographic atrophy (GA) imaged and analyzed on the Zeiss AngioPlex software. The large areas of GA allow the underlying choroidal vasculature to be well visualized.

3.9 Financial Disclosures

P.K.K.: consultant: Carl Zeiss Meditec, Optovue.

References

[1] de Carlo TE, Bonini Filho MA, Chin AT, et al. Spectral-domain optical coherence tomography angiography of choroidal neovascularization. Ophthalmology. 2015; 122(6):1228–1238

[2] Huang D, Jia Y, Gao SS, Lumbroso B, Rispoli M. Optical coherence tomography angiography using the Optovue device. Dev Ophthalmol. 2016; 56:6–12

[3] Jia Y, Tan O, Tokayer J, et al. Split-spectrum amplitude-decorrelation angiography with optical coherence tomography. Opt Express. 2012; 20(4):4710–4725

[4] Kraus MF, Potsaid B, Mayer MA, et al. Motion correction in optical coherence tomography volumes on a per A-scan basis using orthogonal scan patterns. Biomed Opt Express. 2012; 3(6):1182–1199

[5] Chalam KV, Sambhav K. Optical coherence tomography angiography in retinal diseases. J Ophthalmic Vis Res. 2016; 11(1):84–92

[6] Tokayer J, Jia Y, Dhalla AH, Huang D. Blood flow velocity quantification using split-spectrum amplitude-decorrelation angiography with optical coherence tomography. Biomed Opt Express. 2013; 4(10):1909–1924

[7] Rosenfeld PJ, Durbin MK, Roisman L, et al. ZEISS Angioplex™ spectral domain optical coherence tomography angiography: technical aspects. Dev Ophthalmol. 2016; 56:18–29

[8] Huang Y, Zhang Q, Thorell MR, et al. Swept-source OCT angiography of the retinal vasculature using intensity differentiation-based optical microangiography algorithms. Ophthalmic Surg Lasers Imaging Retina. 2014; 45(5):382–389

[9] Wang RK. Optical microangiography: a label free 3D imaging technology to visualize and quantify blood circulations within tissue beds in vivo. IEEE J Sel Top Quantum Electron. 2010; 16(3):545–554

[10] Zhang A, Zhang Q, Chen CL, Wang RK. Methods and algorithms for optical coherence tomography-based angiography: a review and comparison. J Biomed Opt. 2015; 20(10):100901

[11] Stanga PE, Tsamis E, Papayannis A, Stringa F, Cole T, Jalil A. Swept-source optical coherence tomography Angio™ (Topcon Corp, Japan): technology review. Dev Ophthalmol. 2016; 56: 13–17

[12] Topcon Corporation. Swept-Source OCT Angiography: SS OCT AngioTM. Tokyo, Japan: Topcon Corporation; 2015

[13] De Vitis LA, Benatti L, Tomasso L, et al. Comparison of the performance of two different spectral-domain optical coherence tomography angiography devices in clinical practice. Ophthalmic Res. 2016; 56(3):155–162

4 Optical Coherence Tomography Angiography and Neovascular Age-Related Macular Degeneration

Nicholas A. Iafe, Nopasak Phasukkijwatana, and David Sarraf

Summary

Optical coherence tomography angiography (OCTA) and neovascular age-related macular degeneration is an exciting intersection for the retinal specialist. Recent advancements in OCTA technology have resulted in more accurate identification and description of the pathologic microvasculature associated with types 1, 2, and 3 neovascularization. Given the invasive nature of fluorescein and indocyanine green angiography, OCTA is a more favorable imaging modality that provides a more practical approach to monitoring neovascularization at baseline and with sequential follow-up after intravitreal anti–vascular endothelial growth factor therapy. OCTA imaging also has the potential to yield important biomarkers that may be used to guide decision-making for treatment and to glean insight into the pathogenesis of this vision altering disease.

Keywords: wet AMD, age-related macular degeneration, choroidal neovascularization, retinal angiomatous proliferation, choroidal neovascularization, classic CNV, occult CNV, type 1 neovascularization, type 2 neovascularization, type 3 neovascularization

4.1 Introduction

Visual impairment is an important public health concern that leads to a decrease in quality-adjusted life years that is comparable to or higher than the loss associated with chronic systemic disorders such as diabetes, stroke, and heart disease.[1] According to recent population-based studies, age-related macular degeneration (AMD) continues to be the leading cause of blindness in people older than 50 years of age in the developed world.[2] Neovascular AMD, of which there are three subtypes, is the principal cause of severe vision loss in 90% of AMD cases.[3] Advances in the diagnosis and therapeutics of this blinding disorder have served to dramatically improve the management of this devastating disease and will become even more important to accommodate an even greater burden of care due to an increasingly aging population in many countries of the developed world.

Fundus fluorescein angiography (FA), the current gold standard for diagnosing neovascular AMD, is an invasive dye-based imaging modality that requires an intravenous administration of contrast followed by interval fundus photography for at least 10 minutes. FA generates two-dimensional images and provides dynamic information about retinal blood flow. Identification of various patterns of dye leakage, pooling, and staining can aid in the diagnosis of retinal and choroidal pathological lesions such as neovascularization. Though FA can readily identify the superficial retinal capillary plexus, this imaging modality poorly visualizes intraretinal structures such as the deep retinal capillary plexus and the choroid[4] that give rise to neovascular complexes in AMD. In contrast to FA, indocyanine green angiography (ICGA) uses an intravenous dye that enables better visualization of the choroidal blood flow below the retinal pigment epithelium (RPE). During the early stages of neovascularization, however, ICGA may only reveal a hot spot or plaque of fluorescence that is used to infer the presence of an occult neovascular membrane since the morphology of the microvascular complex often cannot be seen. As opposed to FA and ICGA, optical coherence tomography angiography (OCTA) can detect blood flow at various depth-resolved levels of the retina and choroid using an en face platform and provides direct morphological identification of pathological microvascular lesions associated with all subtypes of neovascular AMD.[5,6,7]

De Carlo et al[8] sought to estimate the sensitivity and specificity of detecting choroidal neovascularization (CNV) using OCTA compared to the gold standard of FA. In this study, 30 eyes underwent OCTA and FA for suspected neovascularization on the same date of service. The angiograms were evaluated independently for the presence or absence of CNV. In this cohort, the specificity of neovascularization detection using OCTA compared to FA was high at 91% (20/22), but the sensitivity was low at 50% (4/8). Despite the relatively low sensitivity established in this study, the high specificity indicates that OCTA could potentially be performed as an adjunct to confirm the presence of a neovascular lesion when results from other methods are equivocal.

A study by Inoue et al[9] compared FA and OCTA for the diagnosis of type 1 neovascularization and found comparable detection rates for neovascular AMD between 60 and 70% when either modality was used alone. Added advantages of OCTA included its improved capacity to identify the entire extent of the neovascular lesion and to identify the pattern of microvascular growth. The combined use of OCTA and OCT may provide the most practical and least invasive multimodal approach to best diagnose neovascular AMD.

OCTA imaging also enables quantitative analysis of neovascular complexes over time. Measurements such as area and density of the lesion obtained at baseline and following therapeutic injection may prove to be useful quantitative parameters of treatment response or failure. Other biomarkers of neovascular response are also being investigated including attenuation of the capillary fringe and the presence of flow void areas.[10] The short acquisition time and noninvasive nature of OCTA may provide a more practical modality for sequential imaging in patients with AMD.

4.2 OCTA Features of Neovascular Age-Related Macular Degeneration

Three distinct lesion subtypes constitute the neovascular form of AMD and are best classified according to their spectral domain OCT (SD-OCT) features.[11] Type 1 neovascularization, the most common subtype of neovascular AMD,[12] is identified under the RPE and originates from the choriocapillaris. Type 2 neovascularization, by far the least common of the three entities, is also derived from the choriocapillaris but penetrates the RPE and is therefore located in the subretinal space. Type 3 neovascularization, previously termed retinal angiomatous proliferation (RAP), originates from the deep retinal capillary plexus and is localized in the outer retina. Mixed lesions with features of more than one subtype may also be encountered. Advancements in OCTA imaging will likely result in the development of similar classification criteria based on morphological features of each neovascular subtype.

4.2.1 Type 1 Neovascular Age-Related Macular Degeneration

Type 1 neovascularization, also referred to as occult CNV, originates from the choriocapillaris

and is often associated with an overlying pigment epithelial detachment (PED). It is often difficult to detect an occult type 1 neovascular lesion especially when associated with a PED using standard multimodal imaging consisting of fundus photography, FA, ICGA, and SD-OCT. ▶ Fig. 4.1 illustrates the multimodal imaging findings (color fundus photography, SD-OCT, FA) of macular drusen associated with subretinal fluid, although FA failed to detect a neovascular lesion and only demonstrated staining of the nasal macular drusen. However, OCTA was performed and a treatment naïve type 1 neovascular lesion was subsequently identified. The characteristics of an early or treatment naïve type 1 lesion on OCTA have been described as a tangled web of fine vessels (▶ Fig. 4.1) or a round tuft of small-caliber capillaries in the absence of an associated dilated core feeder vessel.[13,14,15] Roisman et al studied OCTA images of 11 patients with a diagnosis of neovascular AMD in one eye and asymptomatic, nonexudative AMD in the fellow eye.[16] Each patient had previously undergone ICGA on both eyes and the presence of a macular plaque was identified in 3 of the 11 asymptomatic eyes. Subsequent OCTA imaging was able to clearly detect the type 1 neovascular lesion that corresponded to the macular plaques seen with ICGA. Further investigation is still needed to determine the clinical utility of OCTA to noninvasively identify an asymptomatic or early type 1 lesion and to determine the indication for initiation of anti–vascular endothelial growth factor (anti-VEGF) treatment.

Chronic type 1 neovascularization has been noted to exhibit a markedly different morphology compared to early type 1 lesions. The older lesions consist of large, mature vascular complexes with vessels branching from a core trunk composed of one or more large dilated feeder vessels (▶ Fig. 4.2).[5,13,17] This pattern of neovascular growth has been described as a "seafan" or "medusa" morphology. Some researchers have proposed that the dilated core feeder vessels may be the result of chronic anti-VEGF therapy and become more resistant as their endothelial cells acquire protective overlying pericytes. The finer branching vessels at the fringe are primarily composed of unprotected endothelial cells and are therefore more responsive to anti-VEGF therapy.[5,13,18,19] In his seminal paper, Spaide noted the distinction between angiogenesis and arteriogenesis in order to explain the vascular abnormalization associated with chronically treated type 1 neovascular complexes.[13] He theorized that anti-VEGF

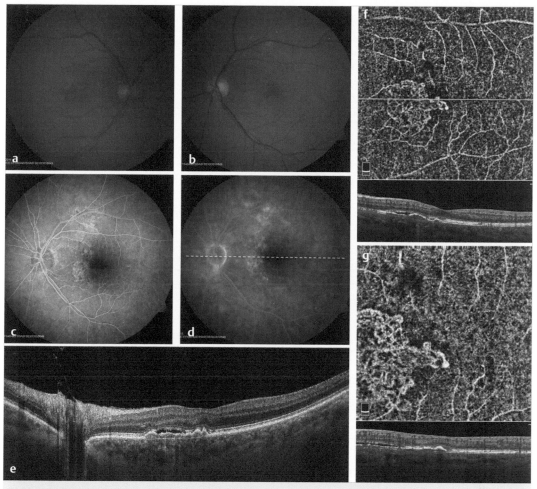

Fig. 4.1 Fundus photographs of **(a)** right and **(b)** left eyes illustrate macular drusen. **(c)** Early-phase fluorescein angiogram (FA) of the left eye shows hyperfluorescence of the macular drusen nasal to the fovea. **(d)** Late-phase FA demonstrates hyperfluorescent staining without clear evidence of dye leakage nasal to the macula. **(e)** Spectral domain optical coherence tomography (SD-OCT) imaged along the yellow dashed line seen in **(d)** illustrates macular drusen or drusenoid pigment epithelial detachment (PED) with overlying mild subretinal fluid. **(f)** A 6 × 6 mm optical coherence tomography angiography (OCTA) and co-registered B-scan. OCTA clearly demonstrates choroidal neovascularization consistent with a type 1 neovascular complex deep to the retinal pigment epithelium (RPE). **(g)** A 3 × 3 mm OCTA with co-registered B-scan shows the tangled web of fine vessels characteristic of treatment naïve type 1 neovascularization. Note that both OCTA images **(f, g)** show projection artifact of the superficial retinal capillary plexus onto the RPE.

treatment leads to the closing of smaller pericyte-poor vessels within the neovascular complex, which results in increased vascular resistance within the lesion. The persistent pericyte-rich vessels remain perfused, however, and are subsequently exposed to higher flow rates and intraluminal pressure, creating a stimulus for arteriogenesis and increased vessel caliber. Cycles of pruning and regrowth of pericyte-poor vessels within a chronic type 1 lesion in response to repeated anti-VEGF therapy causes the mature

pericyte-rich core vessels to progressively enlarge. In the setting of prolonged anti-VEGF therapy, this process can result in the evolution of a neovascular lesion toward subretinal fibrosis.[20,21]

OCTA can also be used to identify type 1 lesions in their late or fibrotic stage. In eyes with subretinal fibrosis complicating neovascular AMD, OCTA often detects blood flow related to recalcitrant vessels located within the fibrotic scar.[22] The vessels in these fibrotic complexes can appear large and dilated with or without vascular loops and

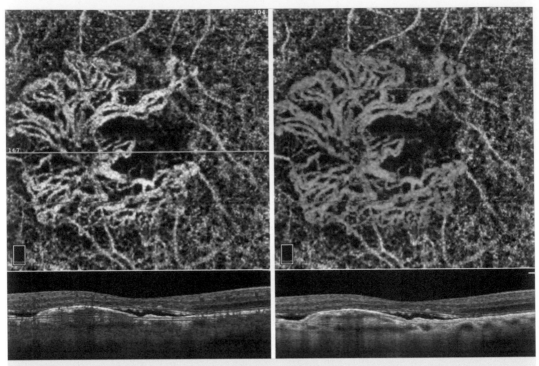

Fig. 4.2 A 3 × 3 mm OCTA (optical coherence tomography angiography) with co-registered B-scan illustrates chronic active type 1 neovascularization (left) and color-coded highlighting of the vessel complex for density analysis (right). Note the large, mature vascular complex with prominent feeder and dilated core vessels and finer interlacing and anastomosing vessels toward the periphery of the lesion.

interconnecting capillaries, but typically consist of predominantly mature vessels without an associated dense capillary plexus (▶ Fig. 4.3). This pattern of neovascular growth has been described as a "dead tree" morphology. The majority of fibrotic lesions also have large flow void areas within the choriocapillaris surrounding the lesion.[17,22] At this stage, OCTA is most useful in determining whether the fibrotic vessels are active or inactive. A proposed set of criteria for evaluating the activity of a neovascular lesion will be discussed later in this chapter.

4.2.2 Type 2 Neovascular Age-Related Macular Degeneration

Type 2 neovascularization, also termed classic CNV (using FA criteria), originates from the choriocapillaris but is located above the RPE in the subretinal space. It is the least common subtype of neovascular AMD occurring in only about 9 to 17% of cases.[12,23] Classic type 2 membranes present as well-defined areas of hyperfluorescence in early FA frames, while late frames demonstrate leakage of dye from the lesion. OCTA images of affected eyes illustrate high-flow vessels above the RPE in the outer retina as well as in the choriocapillaris. The morphology of type 2 lesions has been described as "medusa-shaped" or "glomerulus-shaped,"[24] although the clinical utility of identifying these patterns remains uncertain. These lesions are characterized by oval or globular structures consisting of high-flow vessels entwined with a dense network of finer vessels. Flow void areas are usually seen surrounding the lesion when segmented at both the outer retina and the choriocapillaris. A large feeder vessel is typically identified and may represent the main vessel responsible for piercing through the RPE to give rise to the neovascular complex located in the subretinal space (▶ Fig. 4.4). In rare cases, it is possible to distinguish the afferent and efferent branches that supply and drain the lesion.[25] Concurrent subretinal fluid can also be appreciated with OCTA co-registered B-scans in cases of type 2 neovascularization.

Lumbroso et al[26] assessed the longitudinal progression of naïve type 2 neovascularization following anti-VEGF therapy. In their series of five

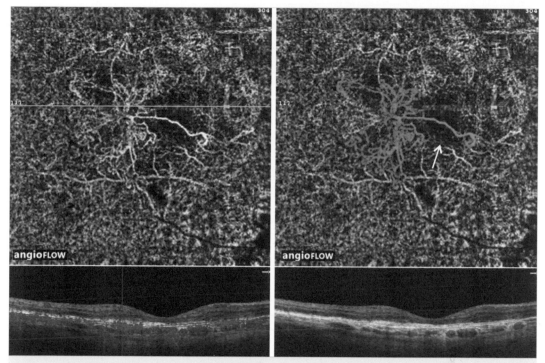

Fig. 4.3 A 6 × 6 mm optical coherence tomography angiography (OCTA) with co-registered B-scan illustrates fibrotic type 1 neovascularization (left) with a long filamentous linear vessel located within the fibrotic scar. The vessels in this inactive lesion appear large and dilated with vascular loops and few peripheral interconnecting capillaries. Also shown is a dark flow void area within the choriocapillaris (arrow) and color-coded highlighting of the vessel complex for density analysis (right). Careful analysis of the full OCTA scan thickness was required to distinguish pathologic vessels from projection artifact seen superior and inferior to the lesion.

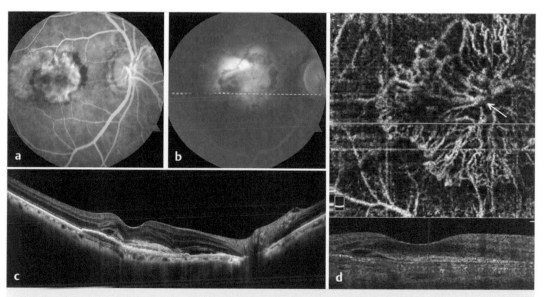

Fig. 4.4 **(a)** Early-phase fluorescein angiogram (FA) of the right eye illustrates a predominantly classic, lacy, and well-defined hyperfluorescent membrane with surrounding hemorrhage. **(b)** Late-phase FA shows leakage of the classic component indicative of type 2 neovascularization. **(c)** Spectral domain optical coherence tomography (SD-OCT) imaged along the yellow dashed line seen in **(b)** demonstrates subretinal hyper-reflective material associated with subretinal fluid and a temporal pigment epithelial detachment (PED). **(d)** A 3 × 3 mm OCTA with co-registered B-scan illustrates a medusa-shaped type 2 neovascular complex located above the retinal pigment epithelium (RPE). The high-flow core feeder vessel (arrow) is the likely entry point into the subretinal space.

female patients, OCTA was performed at 24 hours, 7 to 10 days, 12 to 18 days, and 30 days following each anti-VEGF injection. A predictable cycle of morphological changes was identified at each time point. Twenty-four hours after treatment, OCTA images demonstrated loss of smaller vessels, vessel caliber reduction, and decreased area and vessel density of the lesion as a whole. For the next 7 to 10 days, vessel density continued to decrease, while the remaining vessels with residual flow were observed more prominently near the afferent vessel trunk. Maximal vessel reduction was noted at 12 to 18 days. Twenty-eight to 35 days following anti-VEGF injection, OCTA detected the reappearance of some anastomoses and loops as well as reproliferation of vessels that seemed to be previously collapsed, although the total area of the neovascular lesion remained smaller. These observations seem to confirm Spaide's hypothesis of vascular abnormalization and arterialization that occurs as a result of recurrent pruning of pericyte-poor vessels and subsequent arteriogenesis. Further investigation is still required to determine the clinical significance of identifying morphological changes with OCTA and its potential influence on the timing of anti-VEGF treatment.

4.2.3 Type 3 Neovascular Age-Related Macular Degeneration

Type 3 neovascularization is the second most common form of neovascular AMD[12] comprising 30 to 40% of neovascular lesions in AMD. This entity encompasses two separate terms previously used to describe this form of neovascularization: RAP lesion[27] and occult chorioretinal anastomosis.[28]

Freund et al[29] proposed a new classification scheme of neovascularization in AMD, based on SD-OCT imaging, that was agnostic regarding the origin of neovascularization. Type 3 neovascularization was proposed to represent the intraretinal location of a neovascular lesion. Subsequent studies have shown that these lesions typically originate from the deep retinal capillary plexus.[30] OCTA of type 3 neovascularization has provided persuasive angiographic evidence in support of this origin.[7]

Type 3 lesions are very elusive and difficult to identify with conventional dye-based angiography and even SD-OCT. A subtle "hot spot" with FA or ICGA or only an intraretinal density with SD-OCT may be appreciated.[30,31] OCTA has, for the first time, identified the microvascular morphology of type 3 lesions[7,32,33] and the descriptions have been highly comparable to pathological assessments.[34,35] A small, high-flow vascular tuft of smaller caliber vessels originating from the deep retinal capillary plexus of the outer retina (▶ Fig. 4.5, ▶ Fig. 4.6) has been delineated in several OCTA studies of type 3 neovascularization.[7,32,33] Feeder vessels or retinal–retinal anastomosis can also be appreciated, communicating with the inner retina. In some cases, the type 3 neovascular complex extends posteriorly through the RPE and may be associated with a large PED[30] (▶ Fig. 4.6). Abnormal flow signals corresponding to the neovascularization are also observed within the underlying PED in many cases, although careful analysis is required to distinguish true signal from projection artifact.[33]

In contrast to chronic type 1 and 2 neovascular complexes that tend to horizontally radiate and branch out in a seafan pattern, type 3 complexes

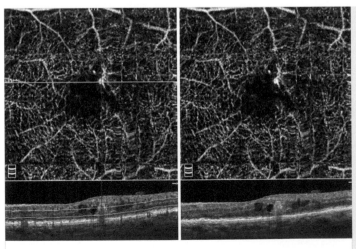

Fig. 4.5 A 3 × 3 mm OCTA (optical coherence tomography angiography) with co-registered B-scan illustrates early type 3 neovascularization with the appearance of a small tuft of vessels originating from the deep retinal capillary plexus (left). Note the flow overlay superimposed on the B-scan that demonstrates emanation of the type 3 neovascular signal from the deep capillary plexus. The B-scan without flow overlay (right) demonstrates intraretinal cystoid macular edema associated with the hyper-reflective type 3 lesion located in the outer nuclear layer, as well as disruption of the external limiting membrane and the ellipsoid zone.

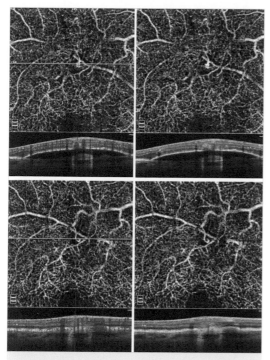

Fig. 4.6 Pretreatment (top) 3 × 3 mm optical coherence tomography angiography (OCTA) with co-registered B-scan illustrates a chronic type 3 neovascular lesion originating from the deep retinal capillary plexus. The B-scans show a large, mixed serous and drusenoid pigment epithelial detachment (PED) associated with a hyper-reflective density that corresponds to the type 3 lesion located in the outer nuclear layer. Follow-up OCTA (bottom) 9 weeks after anti-VEGF (anti–vascular endothelial growth factor) injection demonstrates resolution of the tuft of small vessels and persistence of a bright, high-flow feeder vessel. Co-registered B-scans show reduction in the abnormal flow signal associated with the type 3 lesion and collapse of the large PED.

are most commonly aligned perpendicular to the retinal layers and extend posteriorly to the RPE. Previous authors have attempted to classify different stages of type 3 complexes based on the location and extent of neovascularization, presence of PED and subretinal fluid, and features of outer retinal disruption seen on FA, ICGA, and SD-OCT.[27,28,31] Tan et al[33] used OCTA and co-registered B-scans to study 27 eyes with type 3 neovascularization. Two patterns of flow were observed in this cohort. In pattern 1 (11%), the abnormal flow signal associated with a type 3 lesion was confined to the neurosensory retina. Pattern 2 (74%) was characterized by the extension of the abnormal flow signal through the RPE. In addition, no evidence of

retinal–choroidal anastomosis or abnormal choroidal flow patterns was observed in this study. The authors did acknowledge, however, that the presence of projection artifact beneath type 3 lesions made it impossible to irrefutably rule out the existence of retinal–choroidal anastomosis within an underlying PED. Future OCTA studies with enhanced visualization of structural and flow signals as well as improvements in artifact removal will likely result in a more definitive OCTA-based classification system for type 3 neovascularization.

OCTA can also be utilized to track the treatment response of type 3 lesions to anti-VEGF therapy. Due to the smaller average size of these complexes, angiographic response to anti-VEGF may appear robust as evidenced by the almost complete disappearance of a neovascular complex's flow signal from the outer retina several weeks after injection.[7,32,33] This substantial reduction in flow is very rarely permanent, however, since disease recurrence is the rule. Additional OCTA studies are needed to further explore how different patterns of type 3 neovascularization, response to anti-VEGF therapy, and frequency of recurrence may influence long-term visual outcomes.

4.3 Assessing Neovascular Activity with Optical Coherence Tomography Angiography

The full benefit of OCTA in neovascular AMD will likely incorporate the diagnosis and classification of individual subtypes as well as the assessment of exudative activity in order to guide treatment decision-making. The identification of OCTA biomarkers of neovascular lesion activity has been elusive and awaits more definitive study. While various patterns of neovascular growth have been well characterized using OCTA analysis, indications for anti-VEGF therapy still rely on traditional biomarkers of neovascular activity including the SD-OCT presence of intraretinal or subretinal fluid or the clinical presence of hemorrhage. OCTA promises to provide additional clues of neovascular activity that may further enable the clinician and researcher to better identify and understand the potential of neovascular lesions to grow and their response to therapy, but further research is still necessary to identify these biomarkers.

Coscas et al[10] performed the largest prospective case series to date comparing the findings of traditional multimodal imaging (FA, ICGA, and SD-OCT) to OCTA in 80 eyes with neovascular AMD in order to assess the need for treatment. In this multimodal imaging approach, treatment was indicated if a lesion demonstrated at least two of the three following features: the presence of leakage on FA, evidence of a neovascular network on ICGA, and the presence of subretinal, intraretinal, or sub-RPE fluid on SD-OCT. Each vessel complex was also classified into one of two patterns based on the following five important OCTA findings:

1. *Shape*: well-defined neovascular lesion, lacy wheel, or seafan in shape (vs. long filamentous linear vessels).
2. *Branching pattern*: numerous fine branching vessels typical of a recent lesion (vs. thick, larger caliber vessels typical of a mature lesion).
3. Presence of anastomoses and vascular loops.
4. Presence of a dense vessel termini or peripheral arcade (vs. the absence as in the "dead tree" morphology).
5. The presence of a perilesional hypointense halo that may represent regions of choriocapillaris alteration due to flow impairment, steal, or localized atrophy.

A neovascular lesion was considered pattern 1 (active) if it exhibited three or more of the above features, while pattern 2 (inactive) lesions showed two or fewer features. Using these criteria, there was a 94.9% correspondence between pattern 1 neovascularization and the cases that required treatment based on conventional multimodal imaging. Coscas et al[10] therefore concluded that OCTA could indeed offer noninvasive monitoring of neovascular AMD lesions in order to guide treatment decision-making throughout follow-up.

4.4 Conclusion

Recent advancements in OCTA technology have resulted in more accurate identification and description of the pathologic microvasculature associated with all subtypes of neovascular AMD. Given the cumbersome and invasive nature of dye-based angiography, OCTA is a promising imaging modality that provides a practical approach to more precisely monitor neovascularization at baseline and with sequential follow-up in our rapidly aging population and to more accurately assess responses to therapy. OCTA imaging also has the potential to yield important biomarkers that may be used to guide treatment decision-making and glean insight into the pathogenesis of this vision-altering disease. Improvements in eye

tracking, image artifact removal, and automated quantitative analysis will undoubtedly enhance the utility of OCTA in both the clinical and research arenas.

References

[1] Park SJ, Ahn S, Park KH. Burden of visual impairment and chronic diseases. JAMA Ophthalmol. 2016; 134(7):778–784

[2] Congdon N, O'Colmain B, Klaver CC, et al. Eye Diseases Prevalence Research Group. Causes and prevalence of visual impairment among adults in the United States. Arch Ophthalmol. 2004; 122(4):477–485

[3] Seddon JM. Epidemiology of age-related macular degeneration. In: Schachat AP, Ryan S, eds. Retina. 3rd ed. St Louis, MO: Mosby; 2001:1039–1050

[4] Spaide RF, Klancnik JM, Jr, Cooney MJ. Retinal vascular layers imaged by fluorescein angiography and optical coherence tomography angiography. JAMA Ophthalmol. 2015; 133(1): 45–50

[5] Kuehlewein L, Bansal M, Lenis TL, et al. Optical coherence tomography angiography of type 1 neovascularization in age-related macular degeneration. Am J Ophthalmol. 2015; 160(4):739–48.e2

[6] Kuehlewein L, Sadda SR, Sarraf D. OCT angiography and sequential quantitative analysis of type 2 neovascularization after ranibizumab therapy. Eye (Lond). 2015; 29(7):932–935

[7] Kuehlewein L, Dansingani KK, de Carlo TE, et al. Optical coherence tomography angiography of type 3 neovascularization secondary to age-related macular degeneration. Retina. 2015; 35(11):2229–2235

[8] de Carlo TE, Bonini Filho MA, Chin AT, et al. Spectral-domain optical coherence tomography angiography of choroidal neovascularization. Ophthalmology. 2015; 122(6):1228–1238

[9] Inoue M, Jung JJ, Balaratnasingam C, et al. A comparison between optical coherence tomography angiography and fluorescein angiography for the imaging of type 1 neovascularization. Invest Ophthalmol Vis Sci.. 2016; 57(9): OCT314–323

[10] Coscas GJ, Lupidi M, Coscas F, Cagini C, Souied EH. Optical coherence tomography angiography versus traditional multimodal imaging in assessing the activity of exudative age-related macular degeneration: A new diagnostic challenge. Retina. 2015; 35(11):2219–2228

[11] Freund KB, Zweifel SA, Engelbert M. Do we need a new classification for choroidal neovascularization in age-related macular degeneration? Retina. 2010; 30(9):1333–1349

[12] Jung JJ, Chen CY, Mrejen S, et al. The incidence of neovascular subtypes in newly diagnosed neovascular age-related macular degeneration. Am J Ophthalmol. 2014; 158(4):769–779.e2

[13] Spaide RF. Optical coherence tomography angiography signs of vascular abnormalization with antiangiogenic therapy for choroidal neovascularization. Am J Ophthalmol. 2015; 160 (1):6–16

[14] Muakkassa NW, Chin AT, de Carlo T, et al. Characterizing the effect of anti-vascular endothelial growth factor therapy on treatment-naive choroidal neovascularization using optical coherence tomography angiography. Retina. 2015; 35(11): 2252–2259

[15] Iafe NA, Phasukkijwatana N, Sarraf D. Optical coherence tomography angiography of type 1 neovascularization in age-related macular degeneration. Dev Ophthalmol. 2016; 56:45–51

[16] Roisman L, Zhang Q, Wang RK, et al. Optical coherence tomography angiography of asymptomatic neovascularization in intermediate age-related macular degeneration. Ophthalmology. 2016; 123(6):1309–1319

[17] Coscas G, Lupidi M, Coscas F, Français C, Cagini C, Souied EH. Optical coherence tomography angiography during follow-up: qualitative and quantitative analysis of mixed type I and II choroidal neovascularization after vascular endothelial growth factor trap therapy. Ophthalmic Res. 2015; 54(2): 57–63

[18] Bellou S, Pentheroudakis G, Murphy C, Fotsis T. Anti-angiogenesis in cancer therapy: Hercules and hydra. Cancer Lett. 2013; 338(2):219–228

[19] Benjamin LE, Hemo I, Keshet E. A plasticity window for blood vessel remodelling is defined by pericyte coverage of the preformed endothelial network and is regulated by PDGF-B and VEGF. Development. 1998; 125(9):1591–1598

[20] Bloch SB, Lund-Andersen H, Sander B, Larsen M. Subfoveal fibrosis in eyes with neovascular age-related macular degeneration treated with intravitreal ranibizumab. Am J Ophthalmol. 2013; 156(1):116–124.e1

[21] Channa R, Sophie R, Bagheri S, et al. Regression of choroidal neovascularization results in macular atrophy in anti-vascular endothelial growth factor-treated eyes. Am J Ophthalmol. 2015; 159(1):9–19.e1, 2

[22] Miere A, Semoun O, Cohen SY, et al. Optical coherence tomography angiography features of subretinal fibrosis in age-related macular degeneration. Retina. 2015; 35(11): 2275–2284

[23] Cohen SY, Creuzot-Garcher C, Darmon J, et al. Types of choroidal neovascularisation in newly diagnosed exudative age-related macular degeneration. Br J Ophthalmol. 2007; 91 (9):1173–1176

[24] El Ameen A, Cohen SY, Semoun O, et al. Type 2 neovascularization secondary to age-related macular degeneration imaged by optical coherence tomography angiography. Retina. 2015; 35(11):2212–2218

[25] Souied EH, El Ameen A, Semoun O, et al. Optical coherence tomography angiography of type 2 neovascularization in age-related macular degeneration. Dev Ophthalmol. 2016; 56:52–56

[26] Lumbroso B, Rispoli M, Savastano MC. Longitudinal optical coherence tomography-angiography study of type 2 naive choroidal neovascularization early response after treatment. Retina. 2015; 35(11):2242–2251

[27] Yannuzzi LA, Negrão S, Iida T, et al. Retinal angiomatous proliferation in age-related macular degeneration. Retina. 2001; 21(5):416–434

[28] Gass JD, Agarwal A, Lavina AM, Tawansy KA. Focal inner retinal hemorrhages in patients with drusen: an early sign of occult choroidal neovascularization and chorioretinal anastomosis. Retina. 2003; 23(6):741–751

[29] Freund KB, Ho IV, Barbazetto IA, et al. Type 3 neovascularization: the expanded spectrum of retinal angiomatous proliferation. Retina. 2008; 28(2):201–211

[30] Nagiel A, Sarraf D, Sadda SR, et al. Type 3 neovascularization: evolution, association with pigment epithelial detachment, and treatment response as revealed by spectral domain optical coherence tomography. Retina. 2015; 35(4):638–647

[31] Su D, Lin S, Phasukkijwatana N, et al. An updated staging system of type 3 neovascularization using spectral-domain optical coherence tomography. Retina. 2016; 36(Suppl 1): S40–S49

[32] Miere A, Querques G, Semoun O, El Ameen A, Capuano V, Souied EH. Optical coherence tomography angiography in early type 3 neovascularization. Retina. 2015; 35(11):2236–2241

[33] Tan AC, Dansingani KK, Yannuzzi LA, Sarraf D, Freund KB. Type 3 neovascularization imaged with cross-sectional and en face optical coherence tomography angiography. Retina. 2016:In press

[34] Klein ML, Wilson DJ. Clinicopathologic correlation of choroidal and retinal neovascular lesions in age-related macular degeneration. Am J Ophthalmol. 2011; 151(1):161–169

[35] Monson DM, Smith JR, Klein ML, Wilson DJ. Clinicopathologic correlation of retinal angiomatous proliferation. Arch Ophthalmol. 2008; 126(12):1664–1668

5 Optical Coherence Tomography Angiography and Fibrotic Choroidal Neovascularization in Age-Related Macular Degeneration

Eric Souied and Alexandra Miere

Summary

Optical coherence tomography angiography (OCTA) reveals, in the majority of cases, distinctive, abnormal vascular networks corresponding to the fibrotic choroidal neovascularization (CNV), previously unattainable by fluorescein angiography or spectral-domain optical coherence tomography alone. Three neovascular patterns can be distinguished: pruned vascular tree, vascular loop, and tangled network. Two types of dark areas are also described: dark halo and large flow void. Allowing an in vivo assessment of CNV, OCTA images provide a better understanding of the abnormal angiogenesis occurring in eyes with advanced neovascularization and the evolution process to a fibrotic scar. Moreover, a qualitative assessment of subretinal fibrosis is interesting from a clinical point of view because of the likelihood of new exudative changes within the neovascular lesion, thus demonstrating the potential of OCTA becoming a standard examination for neovascular age-related macular degeneration patients.

Keywords: optical coherence tomography angiography, age-related macular degeneration, choroidal neovascularization, subretinal fibrosis, angiogenesis

5.1 Introduction

Choroidal neovascularization (CNV) is a key component in the pathogenic sequence of neovascular age-related macular degeneration (AMD), leading to loss of central vision over time.[1] While we know today that AMD pathogenesis incorporates a series of factors such as patient age, metabolic dysfunction, oxidative stress, and circulatory disturbances,[2] recent studies have emphasized on the decisive role played by the inflammatory immune response in both the formation and the progression of CNV.[3] Along with geographic atrophy (GA), subretinal fibrosis is a key feature of end-stage AMD.[4] With the advent of anti–vascular endothelial growth factor (anti-VEGF) treatment for neovascular AMD, vision improvement has been possible in 30 to 40% of the patients.[5,6] However,

due to the complex interaction between cytokines, such as VEGF, inflammatory cells, and extracellular matrix in the formation of CNV, the response to anti-VEGF therapy is somewhat limited[7] and the natural history of neovascular AMD ultimately leads to either subretinal fibrosis or macular atrophy, with subsequent poor functional prognosis.

5.2 Subretinal Fibrosis

Subretinal fibrosis is the consequence of complex tissue repair mechanisms and may present either during the natural healing process[7] or during anti-VEGF treatment.[5] Until recently, the imaging of subretinal fibrosis has been based mainly on the combined use of fluorescein angiography (FA) and spectral-domain optical coherence tomography (SD-OCT), which allowed correlation analysis between the angiographic lesion and the corresponding SD-OCT anomaly. On FA, fibrotic CNV is characterized by hyperfluorescent lesions with no leakage in the late frames of the examination, while SD-OCT reveals a compact, subretinal, hyper-reflective lesion, of variable thickness, with possible loss of adjacent retinal pigment epithelium (RPE) and ellipsoid zone.[8,9] Although multimodal structural imaging offers indirect signs of neovessel activity (leakage on FA, subretinal/intraretinal fluid and pigment epithelium detachment on SD-OCT), it does not have the ability to discriminate the various components of a fibrotic scar. The functional outcome of a patient with neovascular AMD could accurately be predicted by differentiating between active neovascular tissue and inactive fibrous tissue.

Optical coherence tomography angiography (OCTA), within the RTVue XR Avanti, with AngioVue software (Optovue, Inc., Freemont, CA) is a new imaging technique that uses the split-spectrum amplitude-decorrelation angiography (SSADA) algorithm to generate amplitude-decorrelation angiography images. Visualization of blood flow allows a detailed evaluation of the retinal microcirculation and neovascular lesions.[10,11]

In a previous paper,[12] we described the OCTA features of subretinal fibrosis secondary to neovascular AMD and compared the findings with those of conventional imaging. The eyes included in the study were classified into two groups, based on FA and SD-OCT findings. In group A were included eyes with evidence of subretinal fibrosis that showed no exudative (subretinal or intraretinal fluid) on SD-OCT over the last 6 months. In group B were included eyes presenting with subretinal fibrosis and recent (< 6 months) exudative signs: subretinal and/or intraretinal fluid, as detected on SD-OCT.

OCTA was able to reveal almost constantly (46 of 49 eyes; 93.8%) a perfused vascular network within the fibrotic scar, with subsequent architectural changes at the outer retina and choriocapillaris levels. In our analysis, three major neovascular patterns, described as pruned vascular tree (26 of 49 eyes; 53.1%), tangled network (14 of 49; 28.6%), and/or vascular loop (25 of 49; 51.0%) have emerged. Furthermore, two types of hyporeflective structures, for which we coined the terms large flow void and dark halo, were observed in 63 and 65% of eyes, respectively.[12] Pruned vascular tree (▶ Fig. 5.1a) consisted of a neovascular network formed by dilated vessels with irregular flow and without any thin capillaries visible when segmenting the fibrotic scar in the OCTA. The pruned vascular tree pattern was present in 50% of study eyes, independently or combined with another pattern. A central feeder vessel was detected in the choriocapillaris segmentation in all cases of pruned vascular tree. Tangled network

(▶ Fig. 5.1b), on the other hand, was characterized on OCTA images by high-flow, interlacing vessels, visible in the segmentation corresponding to the fibrous scar. The third pattern was called the vascular loop (▶ Fig. 5.1c), represented by a convoluted network on OCTA images corresponding to the fibrotic lesion. The presence of two types of dark lesions, flow void and dark halo, could be distinguished in more than half of the study eyes (▶ Fig. 5.2). While the dark halo harbored the aspect of a dark ring in the choriocapillaris segmentation, surrounding the neovascular network (▶ Fig. 5.2a), the large flow void presented as a diffuse lack of signal in the segmentation corresponding to the fibrotic scar, due to masking (▶ Fig. 5.2b).

Two phenotypes of subretinal fibrosis in OCTA have thus emerged: dead tree (comprising lesions with a predominant pruned vascular tree pattern) and blossoming tree, in which tangled network and vascular loop prevail. Interestingly, there was no statistically significant association between groups A or B and a specific vascular pattern or a type of dark area. However, while on FA the original CNV were detected in only 62% of cases, OCTA allowed a much higher detection rate of the underlying neovascular network (93.8% of eyes), offering essential information on the localization, morphology, and perfusion status of fibrotic CNV.

Understanding the way new therapies, such as the anti–platelet-derived growth factor[13] or

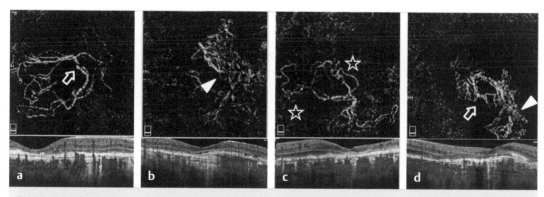

Fig. 5.1 Optical coherence tomography angiography (OCTA) of exudative age-related macular degeneration eyes with subretinal fibrosis: neovascular patterns. **(a)** OCTA image delineates, in the outer retinal segmentation, a vascular network comprising large vessels, with moderately high, filamentous flow (white arrow) and no thinner capillaries visible. The corresponding B-scan shows a hyper-reflective fibrotic scar. **(b)** OCTA images of the outer retinal segmentation and corresponding B-scan show the tangled neovascular network (arrowhead) as a high-flow structure, comprising thin emerging branches and many collateral branches to the surrounding vessels. **(c)** OCTA images of the outer retinal segmentation and corresponding B-scan reveal a high-flow, convoluted network (white star). **(d)** OCTA image and corresponding B-scan show a high-flow, central pruned vascular tree aspect (white arrow) combined with areas of tangled network (white arrowhead) at its terminal part. Adapted from Miere et al 2015.[12]

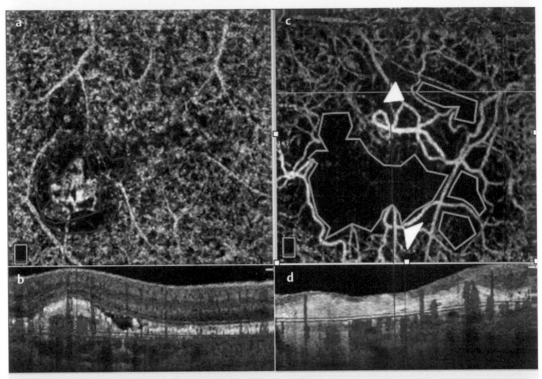

Fig. 5.2 Optical coherence tomography angiography (OCTA) of exudative age-related macular degeneration eyes with dark areas associated to subretinal fibrosis: (**a**) OCTA images at the choriocapillaris segmentation and corresponding B-scan. A tangled neovascular network appears as high flow, round lesion, comprising thin emerging branches. Note the surrounding dark area (red line) surrounding active choroidal neovascularization. (**b**) The OCTA image of the choriocapillaris segmentation and corresponding B-scan show the large flow void as a diffuse lack of signal (blue line), within the high flow neovascular network (white arrowheads)

standard therapies for neovascular AMD, such as anti-VEGF,[5,14] determine morphological changes of CNV, by means of OCTA, could ultimately provide a thorough understanding of the abnormal angio-genesis occurring in eyes with late-stage AMD.

References

[1] Fine SL, Berger JW, Maguire MG, Ho AC. Age-related macular degeneration. N Engl J Med. 2000; 342(7):483–492

[2] Holz FG, Pauleikhoff D, Klein R, Bird AC. Pathogenesis of lesions in late age-related macular disease. Am J Ophthalmol. 2004; 137(3):504–510

[3] Ding X, Patel M, Chan CC. Molecular pathology of age-related macular degeneration. Prog Retin Eye Res. 2009; 28(1):1–18

[4] Zhang R, Liu Z, Zhang H, Zhang Y, Lin D. The COX-2-selective antagonist (NS-398) inhibits choroidal neovascularization and subretinal fibrosis. PLoS One. 2016; 11(1):e0146808

[5] Hwang JC, Del Priore LV, Freund KB, Chang S, Iranmanesh R. Development of subretinal fibrosis after anti-VEGF treatment in neovascular age-related macular degeneration. Ophthalmic Surg Lasers Imaging. 2011; 42(1):6–11

[6] Rosenfeld PJ, Shapiro H, Tuomi L, Webster M, Elledge J, Blodi B, MARINA and ANCHOR Study Groups. Characteristics of patients losing vision after 2 years of monthly dosing in the phase III ranibizumab clinical trials. Ophthalmology. 2011; 118(3):523–530

[7] Kumar V, Abbans K, Nelson F. Robbins and Cotran Pathologic Basis of Disease. 9th ed. Philadelphia, PA: Elsevier Saunders; 2014

[8] Bloch SB, Lund-Andersen H, Sander B, Larsen M. Subfoveal fibrosis in eyes with neovascular age-related macular degeneration treated with intravitreal ranibizumab. Am J Ophthalmol. 2013; 156(1):116–124.e1

[9] Channa R, Sophie R, Bagheri S, et al. Regression of choroidal neovascularization results in macular atrophy in anti-vascular endothelial growth factor-treated eyes. Am J Ophthalmol. 2015; 159(1):9–19.e1, 2

[10] Jia Y, Bailey ST, Wilson DJ, et al. Quantitative optical coherence tomography angiography of choroidal neovascularization in age-related macular degeneration. Ophthalmology. 2014; 121(7):1435–1444

[11] Jia Y, Tan O, Tokayer J, et al. Split-spectrum amplitude-decorrelation angiography with optical coherence tomography. Opt Express. 2012; 20(4):4710–4725

[12] Miere A, Semoun O, Cohen SY, et al. Optical coherence tomography angiography features of subretinal fibrosis in age-related macular degeneration. Retina. 2015; 35(11):2275–2284

[13] Dugel PU, Kunimoto D, Quinlan E, et al. Anti-VEGF resistance in neovascular AMD: role of PDGF antagonism. Paper presented at the Association for Research in Vision and Ophthalmology Annual Meeting; May 2015, Denver, CO

[14] Toth LA, Stevenson M, Chakravarthy U. Anti-vascular endothelial growth factor therapy for neovascular age-related macular degeneration: outcomes in eyes with poor initial vision. Retina. 2015; 35(10):1957–1963

6 Nonneovascular Age-Related Macular Degeneration

Ricardo Noguera Louzada, Mark Lane, and Nadia K. Waheed

Summary

Age-related macular degeneration (AMD) is the leading cause of irreversible blindness in developed countries. Clinically the hallmark of the disease is the presence of drusen and retinal pigment epithelial disruption. As the disease progresses, it can result in geographic atrophy, which can cause significant loss of vision. It is believed that the pathophysiology of nonneovascular AMD may be also associated with a dysfunction in the choriocapillaris. Until recently, evidence for this has been limited to postmortem histological studies. Optical coherence tomography angiography is a relatively new real-time noninvasive technology that generates depth-resolved images of the vasculature of the retina and choroid by acquiring repeated B-scans from the same retinal location. In this chapter, we will highlight how this technology might allow a greater understanding of the pathophysiology of nonneovascular AMD and how it might begin to offer new ways of screening and of monitoring the condition.

Keywords: dry age-related macular degeneration, nonneovascular age-related macular degeneration, nonexudative age-related macular degeneration, geographic atrophy

6.1 Introduction

Age-related macular degeneration (AMD) can cause significant central vision impairment. It is a common cause of blindness in the western world with an estimated prevalence of almost 8.7%. With the aging population, the prevalence is set to increase to 196 million in 2020 and 288 million by 2040.[1]

AMD can be classified into two forms: nonneovascular (dry) and neovascular (wet or exudative). Nonneovascular or dry AMD accounts for 85 to 90% of all cases of AMD. Dry AMD is nearly always bilateral and primarily affects the central area of retina known as the macula. It tends to lead to a gradual but potentially significant reduction in central vision. The visual complications associated with dry AMD increase in severity with age. In the 55- to 65-year age group, only 1% of adults suffer with visually significant disease, compared to 20% in adults older than 75 years.[2]

6.2 Early Nonneovascular Age-Related Macular Degeneration

Early dry AMD is defined clinically as the presence of numerous small or intermediate sized drusen. Drusen are small yellow amorphous deposits of lipofuscin that lie between the retinal pigment epithelium (RPE) and the inner collagenous layer of Bruch's membrane. Drusen deposition is the first clinically visible lesion in patients with dry AMD and is likely to represent the complex disruption of the normal anatomy and physiological processes of the eye.

The choroid is composed of five layers, three of which are vascular: the choriocapillaris (CC), Sattler's layer, and Haller's layer. The CC, the thin capillary layer of the choroid, is located adjacent to Bruch's membrane and has a mutualistic relationship with the RPE.[3,4,5,6] The RPE's function is to provide nutrients and remove waste products from the overlying photoreceptors.[6]

In dry AMD, it is believed that these anatomical structures are disrupted. There is a gradual destruction of the RPE and the photoreceptor layer, thickening of Bruch's membrane, and atrophy of the CC so that the underlying choroidal vasculature becomes visible. There is currently no treatment for dry AMD and it can lead to severe visual impairment.

Several grading systems for the dry AMD exist, with the earliest based on color fundus photography. Of these classifications, the AREDS (Age-Related Eye Disease Study) system has been most commonly utilized to document the site and size of the drusen to help track the progression of the disease over time.[7] Despite fundus photography being readily available, the images only provided two-dimensional data on shape and the spatial location of the drusen and little quantitative data such as change in the drusen volume over time (▶ Fig. 6.1a).

The advent of optical coherence tomography (OCT) has greatly improved our understanding of dry AMD. With the use of high-resolution spectral domain OCT (SD-OCT) and swept-source OCT (SS-OCT), it is possible not only to visualize the individual layers of the retina and the choroid, but to also acquire three-dimensional quantitative assessment of the drusen that are associated with early dry AMD.

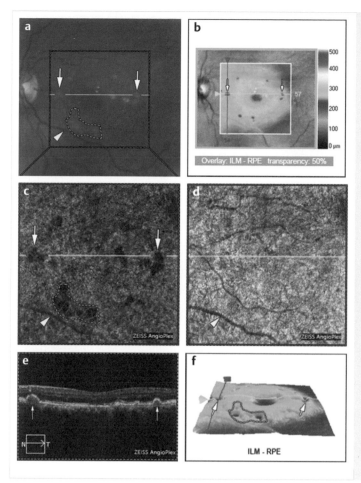

Fig. 6.1 Loss of choriocapillaris (CC) under drusen. CC analysis under drusen using the Zeiss Cirrus HD-OCT with AngioPlex (Carl Zeiss Meditec, Inc., Dublin, CA). **(a)** Color fundus photo; white arrows point to the site of drusen. Yellow dashed line also demarcate the site of drusen. **(b)** Macula thickness analysis. Internal limiting membrane (ILM) and retinal pigment epithelium (RPE) overlay with 50% transparency. White arrows indicate site of drusen. **(c)** A 6 × 6 mm swept-source optical coherence tomography (SD-OCT) angiography CC slab; zoomed in from the fundus photo. Yellow dashed line and white arrows correspond to areas of reduced flow under the drusen. **(d)** The corresponding structural en face scan at the level of CC. There is no loss of signal noted at the site of the drusen, indicating a true-positive flow impairment under the site of the drusen, as noted in **(c)**. **(e)** Corresponding OCT B-scan. **(f)** The thickness map of the corresponding ILM and RPE. There is reduced thickness in the RPE underlying the drusen noted in this figure. The white arrows in **(a–c, e,** and **f)** correspond to the same drusen in each image. The yellow arrow in **(a, c,** and **d)** shows the retinal vessel and its corresponding decorrelation tail (projection artifact).

Drusen are visible on OCT B-scans as hyper-reflective material between Bruch's membrane and the RPE (▶ Fig. 6.1e).[8,9,10] Retinal layers overlying drusen show a thinning in the photoreceptor layer in 97% of cases. It is also noted that the average photoreceptor layer thickness was reduced by 27% when overlying drusen compared to similar sites in normal age-matched control eyes. The inner retinal layers usually remain unchanged. These findings demonstrate a degenerative process with photoreceptor loss leading to visual impairment.[11]

6.3 Optical Coherence Tomography Angiography in Dry AMD

Optical coherence tomography angiography (OCTA) enables rapid, noninvasive, and depth-resolved imaging of the retinal and choroidal vasculature, by detecting the motion contrast from flowing blood.[12,13,14] OCTA images are generated when multiple B-scans are acquired in rapid succession from the same anatomic location. Stationary tissue produces a nearly constant scattering of the OCTA signal, whereas moving tissue such as blood produces an OCTA signal that changes over time. This signal decorrelation is portrayed as a grayscale image where pixels from stationary tissue appear black and pixels from moving tissues appear white. Structural and angiographic datasets can be simultaneously acquired and co-registered, allowing for concurrent visualization of the three-dimensional structure of the vasculature and blood flow.[15,16,17]

Angiography is not a new technique; however, the current gold standard imaging modalities, FA and indocyanine green angiography (ICGA), have inherent flaws in their ability to image the CC. The image quality of FA is reduced by the absorption of

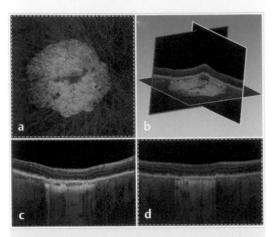

Fig. 6.2 Three-dimensional (3D) view of geographic atrophy (GA) using a 3D slicer. The 3D slicer used was from the free open-source software application for medical image computing available at http://www. slicer.org. The images were acquired using the swept-source optical coherence tomography (SS-OCT) angiography prototype device developed at Massachusetts Institute of Technology (Cambridge, MA). **(a)** En face structural scan of the left eye in a patient with GA. **(b)** Composite 3D image. **(c)** X-fast cross-sectional OCT. **(d)** Y-fast cross-sectional OCT B-scan. Increased penetration is noticed under the GA using the SS-OCT angiography technology. Increased signal penetration occurs under the GA as a result of the retinal pigment epithelium destruction (reverse shadowing). Choroidal vessels are demarcated in red and are clearly visible underlying the site of GA.

the blue-green excitation wavelength of fluorescein by macular xanthophyll and the RPE. The fine microvascular network of the choroid is further obscured by leakage of approximately 20% of the

fluorescein dye that fails to bind to albumin, causing an early hyperfluorescence.[18] Conversely, ICGA, which is considered the superior modality for imaging the choroid, has not gained widespread acceptance as it is not depth-resolved, so separating the CC blood flow from the deeper choroidal vasculature is a complex task.[19,20] In addition, these modalities are invasive, involving the use of intravenous contrast that can result in systemic side effects, such as nausea, vomiting, and, rarely, anaphylaxis.[21,22,23]

OCTA is a noninvasive, nontouch technique and does not require the injection of intravenous dye. This is the key to its use in dry AMD because it means it can be utilized repeatedly in follow-up appointments to track the anatomical disruption of the CC vasculature in patients with early dry AMD as it progresses to late-stage AMD. Despite its huge potential, OCTA is not without drawbacks. OCTA uses volumetric data (▸ Fig. 6.2) to assess blood flow and as such requires increased scanning speeds to acquire this data. This not only increases the time taken to image patients, but also means a reduced scanning field compared to the traditional angiography. This may not, however, be as much of a drawback in AMD where the area of interest is primarily the macula.

En face OCTA permits evaluation of the individual layers of the retina that can be correlated and cross-registered with structural OCT scans (▸ Fig. 6.2b). Using this methodology, it is possible to plot the topological location of the drusen and to compare this with the underlying CC (▸ Fig. 6.1 and ▸ Fig. 6.3). It has been noted that in early dry AMD, some drusen may be spatially related to areas of focal CC loss and that patients with Dry

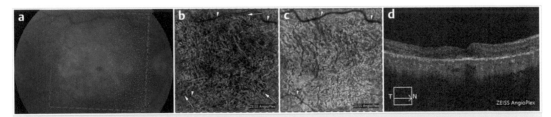

Fig. 6.3 Optical coherence tomography angiography (OCTA) structure of geographic atrophy (GA). OCT Zeiss Cirrus HD-OCT with AngioPlex. Dry age-related macular degeneration and a large central geographic atrophy (GA). **(a)** Fundus photography of the right eye with a large GA. Red dashed indicated the corresponding 6 × 6 mm OCTA. **(b)** A 6 × 6 mm OCTA at the level of the choriocapillaris (CC). There is loss of CC and the larger choroidal vessels are displaced anteriorly occupying the space originally occupied by the CC. The loss of CC underlying the GA is evident by looking between the large vessels (red arrows). Moreover, the CC loss seems to extend beyond the margins of the GA as demonstrated by the white arrows. Yellow head arrows are the corresponding projection artifact from the retina vessels. **(c)** A 6 × 6 mm structure en face OCTA of the GA at the level of the CC. **(d)** Corresponding 6-mm cross-sectional OCT, with the segmentation at the level of the CC.

AMD have a general reduction in CC density compared to age-matched controls (▶ Fig. 6.1c,d). This research is supported by histological data that suggest that drusen often form at the sites of reduced CC density.[5,24,25,26,27] However, since OCTA shows areas of CC void even in normal individuals, it is not quite clear if the changes seen under some drusen represent true CC loss or an incidental intersection of areas of thinned CC with the presence of drusen.

OCTA devices currently fall into two broad categories: SD-OCT angiography and SS-OCT angiography. It is hoped that one of these devices may offer a definitive real-time mechanism for exploring the pathophysiology of AMD. Commercially available SD-OCT angiography devices use a wavelength of 840 nm and have a scanning speed < 100,000 kHz. This hardware has been clinically available for longer and has already been utilized to assess the vascular changes in numerous ophthalmic conditions including exudative AMD and diabetes. However, the shorter, approximately 840 nm, center wavelength used in the SD-OCT systems is strongly attenuated by the RPE. This attenuation can become more severe in the presence of RPE clumping and underlying drusen. Furthermore, the spectrometer-based detection used in SD-OCT is susceptible to so-called "sensitivity roll-off," the reduction in sensitivity at distances further from the zero delay. Both RPE attenuation and sensitivity roll-off can result in low-signal areas in choroidal regions, especially in areas below drusen. It is important to understand the limitations of the shorter wavelength SD-OCT angiography devices, because apparent CC flow impairments under drusen may not be true low flow and may actually be artifact that can be attributed to loss of the OCTA signal.

SS-OCT devices use a tunable laser as their light source and thus offer the potential for greatly increased image acquisition speed. The first commercially available SS-OCT device for retinal applications was the DRI OCT-1 (Topcon, Japan), presenting an image acquisition speed of 100,000 A-scans per second and using a wavelength of approximately 1,050 nm. Recently a new SS-OCT angiography prototype from Zeiss has been developed with 100 kHz SS laser at 1,050 nm. An SS-OCT angiography prototype has been developed at the Massachusetts Institute of Technology (MIT, Cambridge, MA) that uses a high-speed vertical cavity surface emitting laser (VCSEL) as the light source and operates at an approximately 1,050-nm wavelength achieving a speed of 400,000 A-scans per second (▶ Fig. 6.2).

The SS-OCT technology has a lower sensitivity roll-off with depth and allows for better penetration of the RPE, making it better suited for visualizing the choroidal vasculature. This device employs a longer wavelength, which can penetrate further into the CC than the commercial SD-OCT. This improves the visualization of the CC, which can be seen as tightly packed networks of feeding arterioles and draining venules. SS-OCT devices also have a faster scanning speed, which allows for the acquisition of a greater number of volumetric datasets compared to the SD-OCT technology. Since OCTA relies on decorrelation between sequentially acquired OCT volumes in the eye, more dense sampling and acquisition of multiple images improves the information collected for analysis.

Recently, this technology has been utilized to assess the CC under drusen, to try and elucidate the primary defect in dry AMD. It was noted that the longer wavelength 1,050 nm, currently used in SS-OCT angiography, may be less prone to producing areas of false-positive flow impairment under drusen as compared to shorter wavelength, 840 nm, SD-OCT angiography systems. It was also noted in the study that there was not always a clinically discernible reduction in the CC flow underneath all of the drusen (Lane et al, unpublished work). Further quantitative studies must be undertaken to assess if there is a gradual reduction in CC flow that was not possible to elucidate on qualitative grading. A quantitative CC assessment may also offer the chance of predicting patients at risk of developing AMD.

6.4 Geographic Atrophy

Late-stage AMD is a progressive condition that slowly evolves with loss of vision occurring over many years. The hallmark of late-stage dry AMD is the formation of geographic atrophy (GA), which is clinically seen as one or more well-demarcated areas of hypopigmentation due to the absence or destruction of the underlying RPE. These atrophic areas are often accompanied by photoreceptor and CC loss and allow the larger, deeper choroidal vessels to be visualized (▶ Fig. 6.2 and ▶ Fig. 6.3).

Until recently, color fundus photography was used as the standard method to image GA (▶ Fig. 6.3a); however, accurate delineation of the GA outer borders can be challenging, when using this methodology.[28] Other imaging modalities such as fluorescein angiography, fundus autofluorescence, and SD-OCT imaging are now employed to evaluate, quantify, and monitor GA.

The changes associated with GA are easily demonstrable on both SD-OCT and SS-OCT, once the overlying RPE has often been destroyed and will not cause signal attenuation. SD-OCT has highlighted that in GA lesions the outer nuclear layer, the external limiting membrane, and inner and outer segments (IS/OS) junction are gradually destroyed, leading to loss of photoreceptors and CC that can extend beyond the margins of the GA lesion.[29,30,31] However, it is noted that in a smaller number of cases, the CC alterations are only limited to the area of the GA, with no extension outside its limits.[32,33] Evaluation of these junctional zones may provide information about the pathogenesis of GA, and the role of RPE, photoreceptor, and CC loss in the initiation and propagation of this condition.[31]

En face OCT provides numerous advantages, most notably the ability to precisely localize lesions within specific subretinal layers and compare them to the corresponding axial B-scan location. Using this technique, it is possible to visualize the large choroidal vessels that lie below areas of CC loss, in lesions such as GA (▶ Fig. 6.3). En face imaging of the outer retinal layers has been used to help predict the growth of the GA, in patients where photoreceptor loss precedes the progression of GA. In the en face image, the progression of the GA is characterized by the loss of the outer hyper-reflective bands corresponding to the RPE/Bruch's membrane complex and by thinning of the outer nuclear layer with subsequent bunching of the outer plexiform layer toward Bruch's membrane.[34,35] This technique may offer a useful screening tool in the future to help predict patients at risk of progression.

6.5 Varying Interscan Time Analysis

The ability of OCTA to image the CC structure and quantify the level of flow in the CC is the key to the formation of a disease biomarker for dry AMD that will help detect and monitor AMD progression and act as an objective information for treatment responses in clinical trials. Unfortunately, most OCTA techniques have a limited dynamic range and do not provide information about the relative flow velocities within the imaged vasculature.

OCTA devices create flow images by comparing the differences between two consecutive OCT images. If the velocity of erythrocytes in the vessels is very slow, then the two consecutive images that have been acquired may not be sufficiently different for flow to be detected. These areas would appear as areas of no flow even if flow did actually exist. The lowest flow speed that is detectable on an OCT angiography device is known as the "slowest detectable flow" (SDF) and this is based on the interscan time of the device. OCTA devices that are slower have an increased interscan time, and will detect slower rates of flow.

New software called varying interscan time analysis (VISTA) has been created to enable the detection of slow flow and allows the interscan time to be varied depending on the flow rates of the imaged vasculatures. This software takes advantage of the multiple datasets that can be acquired during the same acquisition time due to the faster scanning speed of the SS-OCT angiography machines. Using this software, a comparison between alternate volumetric sets rather than consecutive volumetric sets is made. This doubles the interscan time and improves the sensitivity of SS-OCT angiography devices to slow flow. Combined analysis of both consecutive and alternate scans ensures that slow flow that is missed on consecutive imaging may be visualized when the alternate images are assessed.

VISTA has recently been utilized to show that CC flow impairments exist not only within the GA lesion, but also to a lesser degree beyond their margins. It appears that the CC within the borders of GA tends to be primarily atrophic with no flow, compared to a more subtle flow impairment at margins of the atrophy. The visualization of different flow speeds is an important step toward creating a quantitative OCTA flow measurement and would be especially valuable when assessing diseases in which progression is linked to flow impairment and not just vasculature loss.[36]

6.6 Conclusion

OCTA is a relatively new technique that has the potential to revolutionize the understanding, detection, and monitoring of dry AMD. New techniques, such as VISTA, offer much hope that a quantifiable OCT flow biomarker will likely become available.

References

[1] Wong WL, Su X, Li X, et al. Global prevalence of age-related macular degeneration and disease burden projection for 2020 and 2040: a systematic review and meta-analysis. Lancet Glob Health. 2014; 2(2):e106–e116

[2] Owen CG, Jarrar Z, Wormald R, Cook DG, Fletcher AE, Rudnicka AR. The estimated prevalence and incidence of late

stage age related macular degeneration in the UK. Br J Ophthalmol. 2012; 96(5):752–756

[3] Sarks JP, Sarks SH, Killingsworth MC. Evolution of geographic atrophy of the retinal pigment epithelium. Eye (Lond). 1988; 2(Pt 5):552–577

[4] McLeod DS, Grebe R, Bhutto I, Merges C, Baba T, Lutty GA. Relationship between RPE and choriocapillaris in age-related macular degeneration. Invest Ophthalmol Vis Sci. 2009; 50 (10):4982–4991

[5] Mullins RF, Johnson MN, Faidley EA, Skeie JM, Huang J. Choriocapillaris vascular dropout related to density of drusen in human eyes with early age-related macular degeneration. Invest Ophthalmol Vis Sci. 2011; 52(3):1606–1612

[6] Bhutto I, Lutty G. Understanding age-related macular degeneration (AMD): relationships between the photoreceptor/retinal pigment epithelium/Bruch's membrane/choriocapillaris complex. Mol Aspects Med. 2012; 33(4):295–317

[7] Ferris FL, Davis MD, Clemons TE, et al. Age-Related Eye Disease Study (AREDS) Research Group. A simplified severity scale for age-related macular degeneration: AREDS Report No. 18. Arch Ophthalmol. 2005; 123(11):1570–1574

[8] Moussa K, Lee JY, Stinnett SS, Jaffe GJ. Spectral domain optical coherence tomography-determined morphologic predictors of age-related macular degeneration-associated geographic atrophy progression. Retina. 2013; 33(8):1590–1599

[9] Lutty G, Grunwald J, Majji AB, Uyama M, Yoneya S. Changes in choriocapillaris and retinal pigment epithelium in age-related macular degeneration. Mol Vis. 1999; 5:35

[10] Curcio CA, Messinger JD, Sloan KR, McGwin G, Medeiros NE, Spaide RF. Subretinal drusenoid deposits in non-neovascular age-related macular degeneration: morphology, prevalence, topography, and biogenesis model. Retina. 2013; 33(2):265–276

[11] Schuman SG, Koreishi AF, Farsiu S, Jung SH, Izatt JA, Toth CA. Photoreceptor layer thinning over drusen in eyes with age-related macular degeneration imaged in vivo with spectral-domain optical coherence tomography. Ophthalmology. 2009; 116(3):488–496.e2

[12] de Carlo TE, Bonini Filho MA, Chin AT, et al. Spectral-domain optical coherence tomography angiography of choroidal neovascularization. Ophthalmology. 2015; 122(6):1228–1238

[13] Jonathan E, Enfield J, Leahy MJ. Correlation mapping method for generating microcirculation morphology from optical coherence tomography (OCT) intensity images. J Biophotonics. 2011; 4(9):583–587

[14] An L, Wang RK. In vivo volumetric imaging of vascular perfusion within human retina and choroids with optical micro-angiography. Opt Express. 2008; 16(15):11438–11452

[15] Mariampillai A, Standish BA, Moriyama EH, et al. Speckle variance detection of microvasculature using swept-source optical coherence tomography. Opt Lett. 2008; 33(13):1530–1532

[16] Fingler J, Schwartz D, Yang C, Fraser SE. Mobility and transverse flow visualization using phase variance contrast with spectral domain optical coherence tomography. Opt Express. 2007; 15(20):12636–12653

[17] Makita S, Jaillon F, Yamanari M, Miura M, Yasuno Y. Comprehensive in vivo micro-vascular imaging of the human eye by dual-beam-scan Doppler optical coherence angiography. Opt Express. 2011; 19(2):1271–1283

[18] Bischoff PM, Flower RW. Ten years experience with choroidal angiography using indocyanine green dye: a new routine examination or an epilogue? Doc Ophthalmol. 1985; 60(3):235–291

[19] Flower RW. Extraction of choriocapillaris hemodynamic data from ICG fluorescence angiograms. Invest Ophthalmol Vis Sci. 1993; 34(9):2720–2729

[20] Zhu L, Zheng Y, von Kerczek CH, Topoleski LD, Flower RW. Feasibility of extracting velocity distribution in choriocapillaris in human eyes from ICG dye angiograms. J Biomech Eng. 2006; 128(2):203–209

[21] Ha SO, Kim DY, Sohn CH, Lim KS. Anaphylaxis caused by intravenous fluorescein: clinical characteristics and review of literature. Intern Emerg Med. 2014; 9(3):325–330

[22] Musa F, Muen WJ, Hancock R, Clark D. Adverse effects of fluorescein angiography in hypertensive and elderly patients. Acta Ophthalmol Scand. 2006; 84(6):740–742

[23] Garski TR, Staller BJ, Hepner G, Banka VS, Finney RA, Jr. Adverse reactions after administration of indocyanine green. JAMA. 1978; 240(7):635

[24] Freeman SR, Kozak I, Cheng L, et al. Optical coherence tomography-raster scanning and manual segmentation in determining drusen volume in age-related macular degeneration. Retina. 2010; 30(3):431–435

[25] Lengyel I, Tufail A, Hosaini HA, Luthert P, Bird AC, Jeffery G. Association of drusen deposition with choroidal intercapillary pillars in the aging human eye. Invest Ophthalmol Vis Sci. 2004; 45(9):2886–2892

[26] Sarks SH, Arnold JJ, Killingsworth MC, Sarks JP. Early drusen formation in the normal and aging eye and their relation to age related maculopathy: a clinicopathological study. Br J Ophthalmol. 1999; 83(3):358–368

[27] Sohrab M, Wu K, Fawzi AA. A pilot study of morphometric analysis of choroidal vasculature in vivo, using en face optical coherence tomography. PLoS One. 2012; 7(11):e48631

[28] Sunness JS, Bressler NM, Tian Y, Alexander J, Applegate CA. Measuring geographic atrophy in advanced age-related macular degeneration. Invest Ophthalmol Vis Sci. 1999; 40 (8):1761–1769

[29] Schmitz-Valckenberg S, Fleckenstein M, Göbel AP, Hohman TC, Holz FG. Optical coherence tomography and autofluorescence findings in areas with geographic atrophy due to age-related macular degeneration. Invest Ophthalmol Vis Sci. 2011; 52(1):1–6

[30] Fleckenstein M, Charbel Issa P, Helb HM, et al. High-resolution spectral domain-OCT imaging in geographic atrophy associated with age-related macular degeneration. Invest Ophthalmol Vis Sci. 2008; 49(9):4137–4144

[31] Bearelly S, Chau FY, Koreishi A, Stinnett SS, Izatt JA, Toth CA. Spectral domain optical coherence tomography imaging of geographic atrophy margins. Ophthalmology. 2009; 116(9):1762–1769

[32] Choi W, Mohler KJ, Potsaid B, et al. Choriocapillaris and choroidal microvasculature imaging with ultrahigh speed OCT angiography. PLoS One. 2013; 8(12):e81499

[33] Adhi M, Liu JJ, Qavi AH, et al. Choroidal analysis in healthy eyes using swept-source optical coherence tomography compared to spectral domain optical coherence tomography. Am J Ophthalmol. 2014; 157(6):1272–1281.e1

[34] Nunes RP, Gregori G, Yehoshua Z, et al. Predicting the progression of geographic atrophy in age-related macular degeneration with SD-OCT en face imaging of the outer retina. Ophthalmic Surg Lasers Imaging Retina. 2013; 44(4):344–359

[35] Giocanti-Auregan A, Tadayoni R, Fajnkuchen F, Dourmad P, Magazzeni S, Cohen SY. Predictive value of outer retina en face oct imaging for geographic atrophy progression. Invest Ophthalmol Vis Sci. 2015; 56(13):8325–8330

[36] Choi W, Moult EM, Waheed NK, et al. Ultrahigh-speed, swept-source optical coherence tomography angiography in nonexudative age-related macular degeneration with geographic atrophy. Ophthalmology. 2015; 122(12):2532–2544

7 Optical Coherence Tomography Angiography and Diabetic Retinopathy

André Romano

Summary

Diabetic retinopathy (DR) is a severe sight-threatening complication of diabetes mellitus and the leading cause of blindness in working age in the United States and worldwide. Fluorescein angiography has been used for many years to diagnose and monitor disease severity. Optical coherence tomography angiography (OCTA), however, offers the unique opportunity to study the retinal vasculature using motion contrast to generate blood flow angiograms. As a result, diabetes-related vascular abnormalities can be assessed in a fast, noninvasive manner, including changes of the foveal avascular zone and alterations of the superficial and deep capillary plexus. Since it works with volumetric scans, specific depths, such as the vitreoretinal interface, can be segmented to assess neovascularization. This chapter will focus on the potential applications of OCTA in DR.

Keywords: diabetic macular edema, diabetic retinopathy, microaneurysms, optical coherence tomography angiography

7.1 Introduction

Diabetic retinopathy (DR) is a severe sight-threatening complication of diabetes mellitus and the leading cause of blindness in working age in United States and worldwide.[1] The number of patients affected with this sight-threatening disease is expected to grow as diet and exercise habits, including increasingly sedentary lifestyle, change in developing countries.[2,3]

Pericyte loss, microaneurysm formation, breakdown of the blood–retinal barrier, and capillary nonperfusion impair the nutrition of the neuroglial tissues in the retinal parenchyma, and the resultant hypoxia increases expression of vascular endothelial growth factor (VEGF), which promotes both angiogenic responses and vascular permeability and causes ischemic maculopathy, proliferative diabetic retinopathy (PDR), and diabetic macular edema (DME).[4]

In addition, the diabetic choroid has vascular-related changes similar to those in the diabetic retina. Consequently, systematic evaluations of retinal and choroidal capillaries are essential.

Fluorescein angiography (FA) was introduced in the 1960s as a method for visualizing the retinal and choroidal vessels and rapidly became the gold standard exam for identifying and classifying several of retinal vascular diseases.[5] The method is based on intravenous injection of a fluorescein dye to evaluate retinal vascular capillary network.

Leakage, capillary nonperfusion, vascular structural abnormalities, neovascularization of the disc (NVD), and neovascularization elsewhere (NVE) are among the most common features observed in this technique in a patient with DR. However, this technique is time-consuming, invasive, and while considered harmless, the dyes pose risks ranging from nausea to allergic reactions, including anaphylaxis and, in rare instances, death.[6,7]

7.2 Optical Coherence Tomography Angiography Technique

Optical coherence tomography (OCT) has revolutionized the way we diagnose and treat the structural changes of DR, including macular edema. It provides a three-dimensional cross-sectional view of the retina with micrometer scale-depth resolution.

Optical coherence tomography angiography (OCTA) is a new noninvasive imaging technique that uses motion-contrast imaging by comparing the decorrelation signal between sequential OCT B-scans acquired at the exact same cross-sectional image to generate a blood flow angiogram.

Split-spectrum amplitude decorrelation angiography (SSADA) algorithm is the AngioVue software of the RTVue XR Avanti spectral-domain OCT (SD-OCT; Optovue, Inc., Fremont, CA). It obtains volumetric scans of 304×304 A-scans at 70,000 A-scans per second in approximately 3.0 seconds.[8]

Automated segmentation of superficial and deep inner retinal vascular plexuses, outer retina, and choriocapillaris can be observed in an automated software options of 2×2, 3×3, 6×6, and 8×8 mm OCT angiograms.

7.3 Nonproliferative Diabetic Retinopathy

DR is a microvasculopathy that features increased vascular permeability, microvasculature leaks, and capillaries that are lost early in the disease. Hyperglycemia and mitochondrial and extracellular reactive oxygen species (ROS) are toxic to endothelial cells (ECs), pericytes, and neurons, resulting in their death early in DR.[9]

One of the greatest advantages of OCTA is the ability of scroll through segmented en face slabs across the retinal and choroidal vasculature and therefore may help us to understand the pathophysiology in the course of the disease.

A software preset encompasses four en face zones: a superficial capillary plexus, at the level of the ganglion cell layer; a deep plexus, a network of capillaries between the outer boundary of the inner plexiform layer and the midpoint of the outer plexiform layer (total thickness, 55 μ); the outer retina (photoreceptors), which does not have vessels; and the choriocapillaris (choroid).

The first changes seen in OCTA in patients with nonproliferative DR are vascular remodeling bordering the foveal avascular zone (FAZ), followed by vascular tortuosity, narrowing of capillary lumens, and dilation of its ends. These changes are best seen at the level of the superficial capillary plexus (▶ Fig. 7.1).

Changes in the deep capillary plexus are more difficult to observe due to size and morphology of the capillaries, but with the development of the disease, these modifications may be also appreciated.

This mechanism is explained by EC death from hyperglycemia or leukocyte oxidative burst and subsequent increased vascular permeability appears to occur before pericyte dropout occurs.[10]

OCTA has the disadvantage that it cannot visualize this vascular permeability, whereas FA shows dye leakage from abnormal retinal capillaries.

7.3.1 Microaneurysms

Visualization of microaneurysms is also well delineated with smaller angiograms, but not all microaneurysms are observed in both superficial and deep capillary network, most probably because OCTA is limited by the principle of slowest detectable flow (▶ Fig. 7.2).

The most common microaneurysm morphologic patterns observed in OCTA images are fusiform, saccular, curved, and coiled. Some may have no erythrocytes or blood cells with less motility, which could not be visualized in the OCTA images, although the movement of erythrocytes is not continuous in the microaneurysms.[11]

Some inconsistency in microaneurysms imaging may be found when comparing FA and OCTA images. The explanation may be related to fluorescein dye filling without blood cells or staining of the vascular walls in the microaneurysms, which could be independent of the movement of the erythrocytes.[12]

7.3.2 Macular Edema

Increased permeability of fluid and protein can result in DME. DME is the common cause of visual function loss in both nonproliferative and proliferative DR. These changes depict vascular loops in the presence of cysts in both superficial and deep

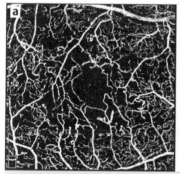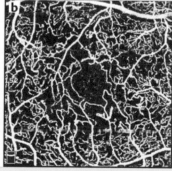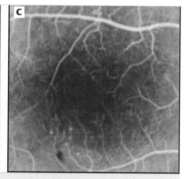

Fig. 7.1 (a,b) Nonproliferative diabetic retinopathy: OCTA shows vascular remodelling bordering the FAZ, capillary tortuosity, narrowing of capillary lumens, and dilation of its terminals adjacent to FAZ at the superficial vascular plexus. (c) These changes cannot be seen in the same manner in fluorescein angiography. FAZ, foveal avascular zone; OCTA, optical coherence tomography angiography.

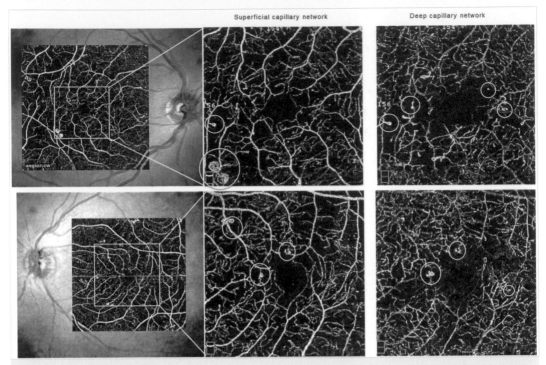

Fig. 7.2 Visualization of microaneurysms is also well delineated with smaller angiograms, but not all microaneurysms are perceived in both superficial and deep capillary networks, most probably because OCTA is limited by the principle of slowest detectable flow. OCTA, optical coherence tomography angiography.

vessels. En face OCT is the best technique to outline cystic changes in DME, and the inner plexiform layer appears to be the best location to appreciate fine details (▶ Fig. 7.3).

7.3.3 Intraretinal Microvascular Abnormalities

Proliferation of retinal capillary endothelium initially causes intraretinal microvascular abnormalities (IRMA), small abnormal vascular formations in areas lacking viable capillaries, which can also be appreciated on OCTA (▶ Fig. 7.4).

7.4 Proliferative Diabetic Retinopathy

Microvascular changes are more severe in PDR. EC proliferation and migration from veins and venules and chronic ischemia can result in the formation of preretinal neovascularization, the hallmark of PDR.

When neovessels are detected on the retina or the optic disc, DR has progressed to the proliferative stage. In contrast to the abnormalities of nonproliferative retinopathy, those of proliferative retinopathy are no longer contained within the retina. Abnormal new blood vessels and connective tissue erupt through the surface of the retina or optic nerve to grow on the posterior surface of the vitreous (posterior hyaloid) or proliferate into the vitreous gel.

Modifying the en face OCTA slab toward the vitreous allows the operator to precisely evaluate extension and morphology of the network without the cumbersome dye leakage and it is particularly useful to pinpoint neovascularization emanating from areas elsewhere in the retina (NVE) or at the disc (▶ Fig. 7.5).

7.5 Ischemic Diabetic Maculopathy

An important hallmark in diabetic macular ischemia (DMI) is tissue hypoxia secondary to narrowing or occlusion of retinal capillaries. It results in an increased VEGF levels and consequently DME.[13]

Furthermore, recent studies have suggested that severe macular ischemia is associated with

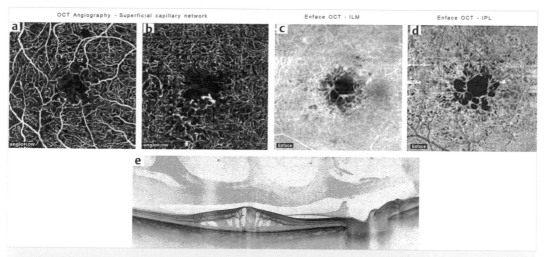

Fig. 7.3 (a,b) Patient with diabetic macular edema. OCTA shows vascular loops and cysts in both superficial and deep plexus. **(c,d)** En face OCT is the best technique to outline cystic changes in DME. IPL appears to be the best location to appreciate **(d)** fine details and correlate it with **(e)** B-Scan OCT images. DME, diabetic macular edema; IPL, inner plexiform layer; OCTA, optical coherence tomography angiography.

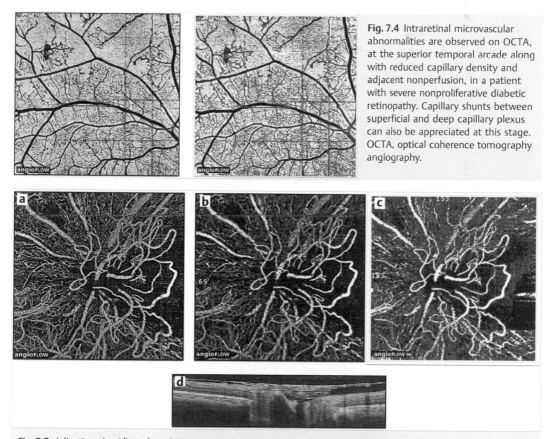

Fig. 7.4 Intraretinal microvascular abnormalities are observed on OCTA, at the superior temporal arcade along with reduced capillary density and adjacent nonperfusion, in a patient with severe nonproliferative diabetic retinopathy. Capillary shunts between superficial and deep capillary plexus can also be appreciated at this stage. OCTA, optical coherence tomography angiography.

Fig. 7.5 Adjusting the **(d)** en face OCT angiography slab toward the vitreous allows the operator to precisely evaluate extension and morphology of the network without the cumbersome of dye leakage and is particularly useful to pinpoint neovascularization at the **(a–c)** disc or elsewhere in the retina.

thinning and disorganization of retinal layers on OCT.[14,15]

FA have shown that FAZ size increases as DMI gravity progresses and is most intense in PDR.[16] However, FA is only able to show the superficial capillary network. On the other hand, OCTA enables us to study both superficial and deep vascular networks.[17]

Following that principle, investigators have shown that FAZ area is larger at the level of both superficial and deep vascular networks in eyes with DR compared to healthy eyes when using OCTA.[18,19] This is also true in diabetic patients with nonclinically detectable DR when compared to healthy eyes.[20]

Nevertheless, these FAZ changes seem to be more accentuated at the level of the deep vascular network and in eyes with PDR.[21] Furthermore, low perfusion is well appreciated and better seen when using a 3 × 3 mm OCT angiogram. It may also depict better vascular details than 6 × 6 or 8 × 8 mm OCT angiogram.

This information may be useful for longitudinal monitoring of FAZ area in DR to track disease progression and visual function changes.

7.6 Quantitative Capillary Perfusion Density Mapping (AngioAnalytics)

OCTA advancement includes the development of different algorithms to quantify FAZ area, vascular density, and areas of nonflow. Recently, an OCTA color-coded capillary perfusion density mapping was developed to discriminate and quantify progressive retinal perfusion changes in DR.[22]

This algorithm, also known as AngioAnalytics (Optovue Inc., Fremont, CA), is based on the conversion of OCT angiogram images from gray scale into a black and white image to improve the consistency and accuracy of perfusion density analysis.

Furthermore, the vessel skeletonization converts the OCTA images to black and white, so perfusion density analysis can be performed for each microvascular layer.

Bright red represents a density of greater than 50% perfused vessels, dark blue represents no perfused vessels, and intermediate perfusion densities are color coded accordingly in the color maps (▶ Fig. 7.6). This analysis can be performed for all three layers in both the 3 × 3 and 6 × 6 mm scans for each subject.

The most significant result of this quantitative color-coded perfusion density mapping comparison between normal and nonproliferative diabetic retinopathy and PDR shows that as disease progresses, FAZ area enlarges and vascular density decreases (▶ Fig. 7.7). The study suggests that patients with

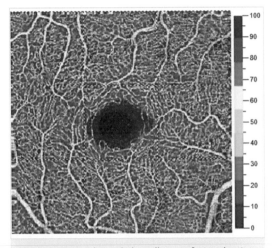

Fig. 7.6 OCTA color-coded capillary perfusion density mapping. Bright red represents a density of greater than 50% perfused vessels, dark blue represents no perfused vessels, and intermediate perfusion densities are color coded accordingly in the color maps. OCTA, optical coherence tomography angiography.

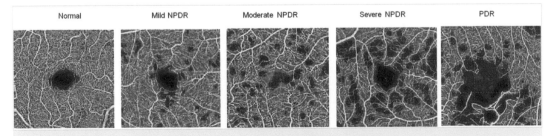

Fig. 7.7 Quantitative color-coded perfusion density mapping comparison between normal and NPDR and PDR shows that as disease progresses, FAZ area enlarges and vascular density decreases. FAZ, foveal avascular zone; NPDR, nonproliferative diabetic retinopathy; PDR, proliferative diabetic retinopathy.

adequate reproducibility at baseline can be monitored reliably over time.[22]

7.7 Conclusion

OCTA has great potential for use in DR because it is noninvasive, provides accurate size and localization information, visualizes both superficial and deep capillary plexus but, most importantly, acquires volumetric scans that can be segmented to specific depths such as the vitreoretinal interface to assess neovascularization.

References

[1] Klein R, Klein BE, Moss SE, Davis MD, DeMets DL. The Wisconsin epidemiologic study of diabetic retinopathy. III. Prevalence and risk of diabetic retinopathy when age at diagnosis is 30 or more years. Arch Ophthalmol. 1984; 102 (4):527–532

[2] Saaddine JB, Honeycutt AA, Narayan KM, Zhang X, Klein R, Boyle JP. Projection of diabetic retinopathy and other major eye diseases among people with diabetes mellitus: United States, 2005–2050. Arch Ophthalmol. 2008; 126(12):1740–1747

[3] Wu L, Fernandez-Loaiza P, Sauma J, Hernandez-Bogantes E, Masis M. Classification of diabetic retinopathy and diabetic macular edema. World J Diabetes. 2013; 4(6):290–294

[4] Aiello LP, Avery RL, Arrigg PG, et al. Vascular endothelial growth factor in ocular fluid of patients with diabetic retinopathy and other retinal disorders. N Engl J Med. 1994; 331(22):1480–1487

[5] Novotny HR, Alvis DL. A method of photographing fluorescence in circulating blood in the human retina. Circulation. 1961; 24:82–86

[6] Kwiterovich KA, Maguire MG, Murphy RP, et al. Frequency of adverse systemic reactions after fluorescein angiography. Results of a prospective study. Ophthalmology. 1991; 98(7): 1139–1142

[7] Musa F, Muen WJ, Hancock R, Clark D. Adverse effects of fluorescein angiography in hypertensive and elderly patients. Acta Ophthalmol Scand. 2006; 84(6):740–742

[8] Jia Y, Tan O, Tokayer J, et al. Split-spectrum amplitude-decorrelation angiography with optical coherence tomography. Opt Express. 2012; 20(4):4710–4725

[9] Zhang X, Zeng H, Bao S, Wang N, Gillies MC. Diabetic macular edema: new concepts in patho-physiology and treatment. Cell Biosci. 2014; 4:27

[10] Tolentino MJ, Husain D, Theodosiadis P, et al. Angiography of fluoresceinated anti-vascular endothelial growth factor antibody and dextrans in experimental choroidal neovascularization. Arch Ophthalmol. 2000; 118(1):78–84

[11] Stitt AW, Gardiner TA, Archer DB. Histological and ultra-structural investigation of retinal microaneurysm development in diabetic patients. Br J Ophthalmol. 1995; 79(4): 362–367

[12] Yeung L, Lima VC, Garcia P, Landa G, Rosen RB. Correlation between spectral domain optical coherence tomography findings and fluorescein angiography patterns in diabetic macular edema. Ophthalmology. 2009; 116(6):1158–1167

[13] Arend O, Wolf S, Jung F, et al. Retinal microcirculation in patients with diabetes mellitus: dynamic and morphological analysis of perifoveal capillary network. Br J Ophthalmol. 1991; 75(9):514–518

[14] Byeon SH, Chu YK, Lee H, Lee SY, Kwon OW. Foveal ganglion cell layer damage in ischemic diabetic maculopathy: correlation of optical coherence tomographic and anatomic changes. Ophthalmology. 2009; 116(10):1949–59.e8

[15] Lee DH, Kim JT, Jung DW, Joe SG, Yoon YH. The relationship between foveal ischemia and spectral-domain optical coherence tomography findings in ischemic diabetic macular edema. Invest Ophthalmol Vis Sci. 2013; 54(2):1080–1085

[16] Sim DA, Keane PA, Zarranz-Ventura J, et al. The effects of macular ischemia on visual acuity in diabetic retinopathy. Invest Ophthalmol Vis Sci. 2013; 54(3):2353–2360

[17] de Carlo TE, Romano A, Waheed NK, Duker JS. A review of optical coherence tomography angiography (OCTA). Int J Retina Vitreous. 2015; 15:1–15

[18] Hwang TS, Gao SS, Liu L, et al. Automated quantification of capillary nonperfusion using optical coherence tomography angiography in diabetic retinopathy. JAMA Ophthalmol. 2016; 134(4):367–373

[19] Samara WA, Say EA, Khoo CT, et al. Correlation of foveal avascular zone size with foveal morphology in normal eyes using optical coherence tomography angiography. Retina. 2015; 35(11):2188–2195

[20] Takase N, Nozaki M, Kato A, Ozeki H, Yoshida M, Ogura Y. Enlargement of foveal avascular zone in diabetic eyes evaluated by en face optical coherence tomography angiography. Retina. 2015; 35(11):2377–2383

[21] Salz DA, de Carlo TE, Adhi M, et al. Select features of diabetic retinopathy on swept-source optical coherence tomographic angiography compared with fluorescein angiography and normal eyes. JAMA Ophthalmol. 2016; 134(6):644–650

[22] Agemy SA, Scripsema NK, Shah CM, et al. Retinal vascular perfusion density mapping using optical coherence tomography angiography in normals and diabetic retinopathy patients. Retina. 2015; 35(11):2353–2363

8 Optical Coherence Tomography Angiography and Arterial Occlusions

Abtin Shahlaee, Carl D. Regillo, and Allen C. Ho

Summary

Microvascular features of branch and central retinal artery occlusion are described using optical coherence tomography angiography (OCTA), and findings are compared with those of fluorescein angiography and clinical examination. OCTA provides depth-resolved information of superficial and deep retinal as well as radial peripapillary capillary networks enabling for assessment of differences in the distribution of reduced vascular flow in the setting of retinal artery occlusive disease. In this regard, OCTA also provides further insight into the pathogenesis of paracentral acute middle maculopathy. Overall, OCTA can be used for diagnosis and monitoring changes in vascular flow during the clinical course of retinal artery occlusion.

Keywords: optical coherence tomography, angiography, retinal artery occlusion, imaging

8.1 Overview of Vascular Anatomy

Central retinal artery occlusion (CRAO) presents as sudden, catastrophic visual loss and is therefore, one of the most important topics in ophthalmology. Similarly, branch retinal arterial, or better termed arteriolar, occlusion (BRAO) causes sudden segmental visual loss that may recur to involve other branch retinal arterioles. The incidence of CRAO has been estimated to be 1 to 10 in 100,000.[1] Symptomatic BRAO is even less common. Yet, acute retinal arterial occlusions (RAOs) are among the major causes of acute visual loss. Accurate and timely diagnosis of RAO is critical because permanent retinal damage may ensue by 4 hours following the initial ischemic insult.[2] Additionally, visual deficits may be the initial presenting sign in individuals at risk of morbidity from systemic embolic events.

The arterial blood supply to the retina and choroid is composed of two main systems both derived from the ophthalmic artery. The ophthalmic artery is the first branch of the internal carotid artery and enters the orbit through the optic canal below the optic nerve. The central retinal artery (CRA), the primary source of blood supply to the retina, is the first intraorbital branch of the ophthalmic artery that passes into the optic nerve at 8 to 15 mm behind the globe to provide the blood supply to the inner retina.[2] The outer retina and choroid receive blood supply from the short posterior ciliary arteries (PCAs) that branch distally from the ophthalmic artery. The main branches of the CRA course horizontally throughout the superficial nerve fiber layer (NFL), intermittently diving into the deeper layers. From their terminal arterioles and venules, precapillary and capillary tributaries sprout nearly perpendicular to the retinal surface, bending into the deeper retinal layers where they anastomose laterally to form distinct microvascular capillary systems. The superficial system resides predominantly within the NFL and ganglion cell layer. Approaching the optic disc, the NFL component is more prominent and the capillary bed is referred to as the radial peripapillary capillary (RPC) plexus, but as it moves toward the fovea, these vessels predominantly localize within the ganglion cell layer and are referred to as the superficial capillary plexus (SCP). The RPC plexus plays an important role in the development of several lesions such as cotton wool spots (CWS) that are often located along its distribution.[2] The deeper system is composed of an intermediate capillary plexus (ICP) and a deep capillary plexus (DCP) located at the inner and outer planes of the inner nuclear layer (INL), respectively. Consequently, in the region of the central macula, an intricate array of capillary networks exists within a superficial, intermediate, and deep trilaminar system that are interconnected by perpendicularly oriented diving vessels. It has been proposed that these individual layers of the retinal vasculature may be differentially affected by ischemic retinal vascular disease.[3]

Notably, the foveola receives its blood supply from the choroidal circulation and is not supplied by the CRA or its branches. An important anatomical variation among 15 to 20% of the population is the presence of a cilioretinal artery that usually arises from the peripapillary choroid or directly from one of the short PCAs. The cilioretinal artery has a characteristic hooklike appearance at its site of entry into the retina at the optic disc margin, usually on the temporal side and less frequently elsewhere. The size and area of the retina supplied by a cilioretinal artery vary widely from a minute artery supplying a small area of the peripapillary retina to supplying half or even the entire retina.[2] When present, the cilioretinal artery may provide additional blood supply to the retina, including the nerve fibers from the foveal photoreceptors, which could result in areas of preserved central vision in cases of central retina artery occlusion (CRAO) as demonstrated in ▸ Fig. 8.1. However, it is also possible for the cilioretinal artery to occlude in

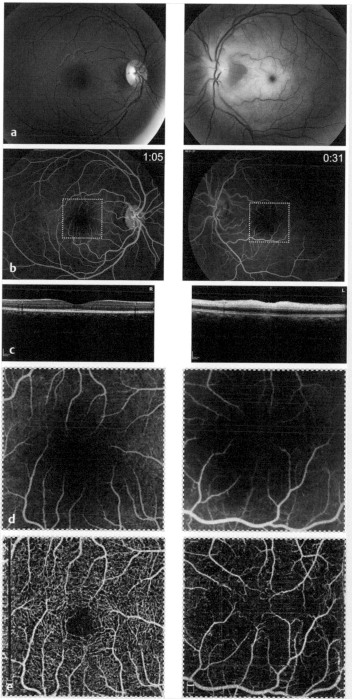

Fig. 8.1 Multimodal imaging of acute central retinal arterial occlusion in a 24-year-old female with light perception in the left eye and 20/40 vision in the fellow eye. Left column shows affected eye and right column represents normal fellow eye. Color fundus photograph demonstrates retinal whitening with a "cherry-red spot" at the (a) foveola. Note the spared area nasal to optic nerve perfused by the cilioretinal artery. Fluorescein angiography (FA) demonstrated delayed transit and late hyperfluorescence consistent with (b) macular edema and increased thickness on (c) optical coherence tomography (OCT). Furthermore, decreased arterial perfusion is evident in the macula (yellow dashed region) on FA by comparing areas of hypofluorescence to the (d) fellow eye. OCT angiography of similar regions demonstrates flow void with more capillary detail. This further enables enhanced visualization of the (e) foveal avascular zone.

isolation, causing central visual field loss with a perfused macula region.

8.2 Pathogenesis and Diagnosis

BRAO usually results from embolic obstruction of a division of the retinal artery, while CRAO results from occlusion of the retinal artery before it branches either at or proximal to the optic disc. CWSs are common, acute, nonspecific retinal lesions, seen in retinopathies due to a whole host of conditions. They are the result of occlusion of the terminal retinal arterioles in the nerve fiber and ganglion cell layer, with focal nonperfusion of the retinal capillaries in their distribution, resulting in acute focal inner retinal ischemia and infarction.[2] Individuals with RAO typically present with unilateral, painless sudden loss of vision or scotoma due to interruption of the blood supply to the retina. Acute obstruction of the retinal artery with subsequent collapse of capillary flow leads to axoplasmic stasis, intracellular edema, and ischemic necrosis of the inner retinal layers. This causes opacification of the NFL and inner retina, creating a glassy and whitened appearance within 15 minutes to several hours following the injury. This opacification is densest at the posterior pole, given the macular region, unlike the rest of the retina, has more than one layer of retinal ganglion cells, and it is the thickest part of the retina.[2] The foveola assumes a "cherry-red spot" appearance because it remains nourished from the choroidal circulation, and thus, the retinal pigment epithelium and choroid remain intact underneath the fovea, while the surrounding retina opacifies (▶ Fig. 8.1). If the CRA becomes occluded, complete loss of vision occurs even though the central foveolar circulation is not affected owing to ischemia of the emanating NFL. Pigmentary changes are usually absent because the retinal pigment epithelium remains unaffected. The blood column in both the arteries and the veins can become segmented with separation of serum from Rouleau stacking of the red corpuscles leading to a "box-carring" appearance (▶ Fig. 8.2). The clinical appearance of retinal whitening resolves in 4 to 6 weeks over which course the obstructed retinal artery will usually recanalize and reperfuse with resolution of the edema. Nonetheless, the inner retinal damage is permanent, leading to atrophy, retinal vascular attenuation, and optic nerve pallor. Hence, visual acuity and/or field loss often do not recover after RAO, given the retinal damage becomes established rapidly with no effective way to reverse the obstruction. Conventional advocate treatments consist of ocular massage to dislodge a CRA embolus, reduction of intraocular pressure by various medical and surgical means to increase retinal perfusion pressure, vasodilation of the CRA by sublingual isosorbide dinitrate, rebreathing of expired CO_2 in a bag, or breathing carbogen or retrobulbar vasodilators, antiplatelet therapy, and heparin therapy.

Establishing a clinical diagnosis of RAO is usually not difficult during the acute phase when retinal whitening and blood flow/vascular alterations are evident on examination. However, these signs may not be obvious very early in the course of disease, in eyes with partial RAO or several weeks after onset. Ancillary imaging studies consisting of intravenous fluorescein angiography (FA) and spectral-domain optical coherence tomography (SD-OCT) are useful to evaluate the presence and extent of retinal nonperfusion, foveal contour, and macular edema, to search for other vascular abnormalities, and to determine the presence or location of retinal emboli. Imaging may also be useful in atypical cases or if acute signs are not apparent. In the acute setting, FA delineates the extent of retinal involvement, seen as capillary nonperfusion and absent or delayed filling of the blood vessels distal to the obstruction. It specifically shows delays in both the arteriovenous transit time and retinal arterial filling with normal choroidal filling. Ophthalmic artery or carotid artery obstruction should be considered if there is delayed choroidal filling. In the chronic setting, FA may show arterial narrowing with normal fluorescein transit following resolution and recanalization of RAO. FA mainly provides information about large vessel flow and SCP but does not allow for assessment of the morphology of the DCP or RPC. In addition, assessment of the deeper retinal capillaries with FA may further be limited by light scattering from the opacified inner retinal layers.[4] SD-OCT can be utilized to determine the specific retinal level of edema or subsequent atrophy during the chronic phase, when FA may no longer display any perfusion deficit.

Optical coherence tomography angiography (OCTA) may have advantages over other imaging techniques. It enables three-dimensional and en face visualization of flow across desired slabs through the retinal and choroidal vasculature. Thus, it can reveal deficiencies involving acute flow interruption in RAO. In addition, it provides en face segmented imaging of the DCP and RPC, which are poorly imaged with FA, and reveals finer details of the SCP.[5] Precise localization of retinal capillary ischemia with OCTA in RAO may help determine subsequent visual prognosis.[2,4] Furthermore, it is

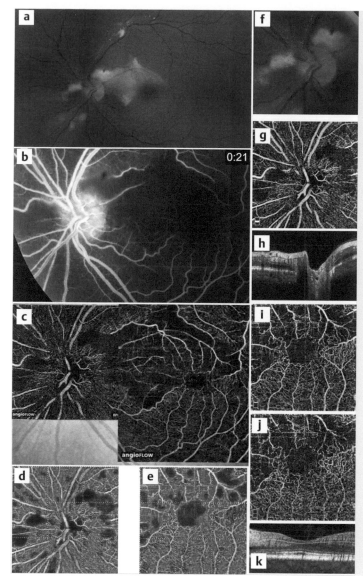

Fig. 8.2 Multimodal imaging of acute branch retinal arterial occlusion in a 60-year-old female. Visual acuity was 20/40 in both eyes. However, the patient complained of a field defect in her left eye. (a) Fundus photo demonstrates multiple cotton wool spots along with retinal whitening, box-carring or cattle-trucking of flow and refractile lesions within the blood vessels. (b) Fluorescein angiography and (c) optical coherence tomography angiography at the (g) radial peripapillary capillary, and (i) superficial and (j) deep capillary plexus levels outline regions of decreased perfusion that correspond to (a,f) retinal whitening. B-scans through the areas of nonperfusion reveal absence of flow signal over areas of (h, k) hyper-reflectivity. Color-coded perfusion maps show the extent of (d,e) involvement.

noninvasive utilizing motion contrast and obviating the need for injectable dyes. This is especially beneficial for patients with concomitant medical problems who may not be able to tolerate dye-based angiography.

8.3 Features of Arterial Occlusion on Optical Coherence Tomography Angiography

▶ Fig. 8.1 demonstrates a case of CRAO with a typical "cherry-red spot" and notable cilioretinal

artery perfusion on clinical examination. FA and OCTA images have been compared to one another and between fellow eyes outlining areas of nonperfusion and demonstrating finer capillary details using OCTA. A case of acute BRAO is presented in ▶ Fig. 8.2. The retinal capillary nonperfusion is more easily discernable on OCTA than on FA. In addition to providing detailed imaging of perfusion status, the coregistered B-scans can also be used to assess retinal thickness and macular edema. Individual assessment of RPC, SCP, and DCP is also possible. Together, these allows for more accurate evaluation of the level and extent of

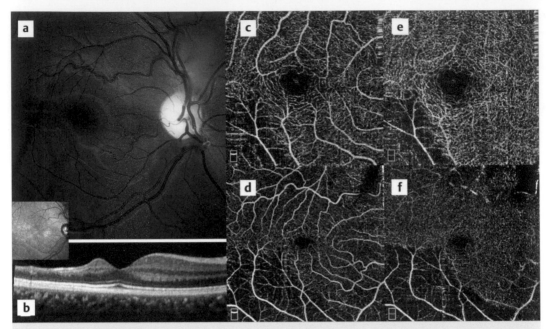

Fig. 8.3 (a) Optical coherence tomography angiography (OCTA) of chronic branch retinal artery occlusion in an 18-year-old male with a prepapillary vascular loop. (b) Radial B-scan reveals inner retinal atrophy inferotemporal to the macula. OCTA shows decreased capillary perfusion in both retinal capillary networks on 3 × 3 and 6 × 6 mm scans. The extent of capillary nonperfusion appears less in the (c, d) superficial capillary network slabs compared to the (e, f) deep. Furthermore, arteries and arterioles remain perfused over areas of ischemia.

involvement in the setting of arterial occlusions. Examples of such differential perfusion have been presented in a case of chronic BRAO (► Fig. 8.3) and CWS (► Fig. 8.4).

FA utilizes the dynamic properties of blood flow to show the early and late changes in retinal vasculature. However, it is limited in imaging only the SCP. In the setting of vascular occlusions, the dynamic nature of the fluorescein images is not essential to making the diagnosis. As seen in ► Fig. 8.1, the resolution of FA is limited and, although it is able to show some areas of capillary nonperfusion, it does not demonstrate subtle microvascular alterations such as the foveal avascular zone alterations. In comparison, OCTA provides flow information at a fixed time point. OCTA enables improved visualization of the retinal microvasculature with more precise demarcation of nonperfusion, which is depth-resolved by segmentation into individual vascular plexuses. By segmentation anterior to Bruch's membrane, the choroidal vasculature can be omitted from the OCTA images, whereas the choroidal flush is seen in FA images, making it harder to discern areas of retinal capillary nonperfusion. This aids in

visualizing subtle vascular changes and may prove useful to quantify and further localize the foci of retinal ischemia in retinal artery occlusive disorders. The ability of OCTA to visualize fine microvascular changes may also allow for the early detection of neovascularization or anastomoses that may arise as a consequence of vascular occlusion.

There have been several recent reports describing microvascular changes in retinal arterial occlusions using OCTA.[4,6,7] In a series of three eyes with CRAO and four eyes with BRAO, Bonini Filho et al[4] found distinct differences in the distribution of zones of decreased vascular perfusion between the superficial and deep retinal capillary plexus corresponding to areas of delayed dye perfusion on FA, suggesting that OCTA imaging can accurately discern retinal capillary plexuses at different levels in the eyes with arterial occlusion and may be sensitive for more precisely characterizing the extent of macular ischemia and monitoring vascular flow changes during the course of the disease. In this series, eyes with acute CRAO demonstrated equal areas of decreased vascular perfusion in both the SCP and DCP, while one eye with CRAO and cilioretinal sparing revealed a wider area of decreased

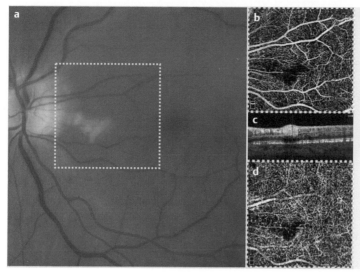

Fig. 8.4 Optical coherence tomography angiography of a **(a)** cotton wool spot demonstrating capillary flow void at the **(b)** superficial vascular network. B-scan demonstrates decreased flow signals over areas of **(c)** nerve fiber layer involvement. The area of decreased perfusion appears smaller in the **(d)** deep capillary plexus.

vascular perfusion in the SCP compared to the DCP. In four eyes with BRAO, 75% of the eyes had a larger area of decreased vascular perfusion in the SCP compared to the DCP, while one eye showed a wider area of decreased vascular perfusion in the deep network. During the chronic phase of RAO, re-established flow was observed in some retinal arterioles on OCTA. Bonini Filho et al hypothesized that reorganization of vascular interconnections in chronic RAO may contribute to partial restoration of DCP perfusion in regions where the SCP remains abnormal. However, caution should be taken when evaluating deep retinal capillary network flow because there may be an element of signal attenuation secondary to inner retinal layer optical reflectivity-producing artifacts masking as hypoperfusion. On the other hand, increased reflectivity of the deeper retinal layers may pronounce the amount of projection artifact from the superficial flow falsely increasing the flow signal seen on the en face image.[8] Therefore, assessment of coregistered OCT B-scans and projection tails may assist in the evaluation of segmentation errors and projection artifacts. Furthermore, OCTA may not always enable differentiation between the superficial and deep retinal networks due to extreme inner retinal thinning secondary to the chronic phase after RAO. OCTA images of the optic disc have been used to evaluate the RPC network in eyes with RAO with variable findings.[4] In CRAO, either preservation or diffuse attenuation of the RPC system has been observed. Eyes with BRAO have demonstrated focal attenuation of the RPCs distributed in the affected arterial occlusion.

Overall, OCTA in RAO reveals varying degrees of vascular nonperfusion in the superficial versus the deep retinal capillary network. This finding is in agreement with the results of SD-OCT B-scan studies demonstrating a spectrum of capillary ischemia in retinal artery occlusive disease, ranging from isolated to continuous superficial and/or deep capillary ischemia.[9] It is not clear what factors affect the variations in the location and severity of nonperfusion/ischemia in RAO. One hypothesis is that inner retinal edema during the early stages of RAO causes compression of the ganglion cell and NFLs, potentially leading to more severe nonperfusion of the SCP. Future studies may shed more light on the determining factors affecting the level of retinal ischemia in RAO.

8.4 Deep Capillary Ischemia

Use of OCTA and coregistered en face structural OCT images has expanded our knowledge about deep capillary ischemia in subjects with paracentral acute middle maculopathy (PAMM). PAMM is a recently described entity in patients presenting with an acute-onset paracentral scotoma. SD-OCT findings include hyper-reflective bandlike lesions at the level of the INL.[10] Although these acute lesions resolve, corresponding atrophy of the INL, resulting in a permanent paracentral visual field defect, ensues, suggesting an INL infarct. It is thought that deep retinal capillary ischemia is the causative factor for the development of these lesions, given the ICP and DCP flank the inner and outer boundaries of the INL, respectively. However,

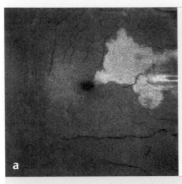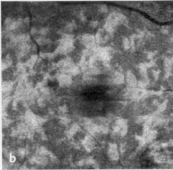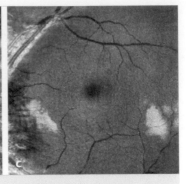

Fig. 8.5 Patterns of paracentral acute middle maculopathy observed on deep slab en face optical coherence tomography. Based on the vascular levels of involvement there may be **(a)** arteriolar, **(b)** perivenular, and **(c)** focal globular distribution of hyper-reflectivity.

definitive evidence of the ischemic origin of PAMM has been lacking. With OCTA, it is possible to obtain high-resolution, depth-resolved en face structural and also functional images of the retinal microvasculature, including the DCP. Hence, subclinical macular lesions of PAMM, which were formerly best visualized on near-infrared reflectance imaging, with SD-OCT hyper-reflectivity can be localized and outlined more precisely using en face OCT. In this regard, we recently proposed a classification scheme and corresponding hypothetical pathophysiological mechanisms for PAMM based on en face patterns.[11] Accordingly, the following three patterns were described that could be present individually or in combination: arteriolar, fernlike, and globular (▶ Fig. 8.5). The arteriolar pattern was observed most commonly and showed bandlike hyper-reflectivity corresponding to the distribution of a large retinal arteriole, and is thought to be caused by either transient or true arteriolar occlusion. The fernlike pattern was seen in the setting of retinal vein occlusion with multifocal parafoveal middle retina hyper-reflectivity due to perivenular ischemia. The globular pattern showed either a focal ovoid patch or multifocal ovoid patches of middle retina hyper-reflectivity caused by distal pericapillary or capillary ischemia.

Furthermore, several reports have looked into perfusion status of PAMM lesions showing preservation of perfusion in focal acute lesions and pruning of the DCP in old cases.[11,12,13,14,15,16] Hence, it has been hypothesized that the pathogenesis of PAMM may be related to ischemia-reperfusion injury under select circumstances, accounting for the persistent capillary flow in some focal acute PAMM lesions and the subsequent legacy of

atrophy of the INL associated with loss of the DCP. In cases with diffuse acute PAMM lesions occurring in the setting of CRAO, that is, large vessel obstruction, capillary reperfusion may never occur, causing severe acute impairment of flow within the DCP[14] as demonstrated in ▶ Fig. 8.6. OCTA of these lesions acutely demonstrates decreased perfusion within the DCP. The hyper-reflective bandlike lesions of the INL characteristic of PAMM in the acute setting eventually resolve over weeks, and corresponding thinning of the INL ensues, indicative of old PAMM lesions or old INL infarcts. OCTA during this chronic phase demonstrates loss of flow within the DCP. Patchy flow voids may be identified within the DCP, and evidence of projection artifacts may be detected from the overlying SCP.[8,14] It has also been proposed that the extent of DCP dropout on OCTA may reflect the extent of visual acuity impairment.[16]

8.5 Limitations

There are several challenges for utilizing OCTA in its current form. There may be technical limitations in obtaining gradable images from individuals with advanced age, long axial length, significant movement, poor fixation, or poor cooperation, and many of these conditions may be present in subjects with retinal vascular disease. In a series of normal eyes, in spite of obtaining reproducible images, we found that 18% of subjects did not fulfill the criteria set for acceptable image quality.[17] This number could potentially be higher in subjects with pathology. Nonetheless, there are currently limited resources for evaluating reproducibility of findings, and comparing normal

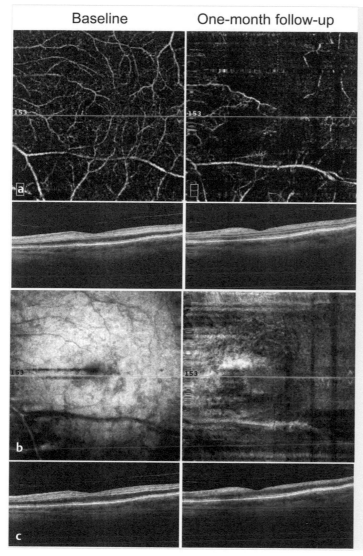

Baseline — **One-month follow-up**

Fig. 8.6 A case of diffuse paracentral acute middle maculopathy secondary to a central retinal artery occlusion. Mildly decreased **(a)** deep capillary perfusion and diffuse middle layer hyper-reflectivity is notable on **(b)** en face and **(c)** cross-sectional imaging on acute presentation. On 1-month follow-up, profound hypoperfusion and hyporeflectivity are seen in the same slab due to development of inner nuclear layer atrophy.

age-matched subjects to those with ocular disease as OCTA technology is relatively new in the clinical setting. A further limitation of OCTA is that the current autosegmentation does not separate the ICP from the DCP, and qualitative and functional distinction requires customized segmentation.[18] In addition, in the setting of arterial occlusions there are often structural and optical reflectivity changes resulting from edema and/or atrophy that may affect the accuracy of en face segmentation and amount of projection of superficial flow. Additionally, the structural and optical reflectivity changes during the course of disease make inter-visit comparison challenging. While this may limit

assessment of individual retinal capillary networks, using the summed en face image of the entire inner retina may still provide useful information that parallels FA findings.[4] Limited field of view is a further shortcoming as the affected area may well extend beyond that of the small OCTA scanning areas. At present, increasing the size of the area scanned reduces the OCTA flow details. Creating montage images of multiple 3 × 3 mm scans has been employed manually to provide a wider field of view while maintaining microvascular detail[19] but is time-consuming and not applicable to a busy clinical setting. Wide-field OCTA is an area currently being explored;[20] the ability to scan larger areas of the retina with high resolution or to montage multiple scans may become an automatic feature in future OCTA technology. Future advances in OCTA imaging permitting an increased scanning area, a reduction in motion and projection artifacts,[21] adjustment for reflectivity of retinal layers, employment of eye tracking, improved segmentation, and a decreased image acquisition time may improve the accuracy of microvasculature imaging in retinal vascular disease. Furthermore, carefully designed studies are required to develop normative reference standards, to which findings in disease can be compared and to validate this imaging technique for appropriate use in clinical practice.

8.6 Conclusion

OCTA may be a sensitive tool to assess the extent of macular ischemia and monitor vascular flow changes during the course of retinal vascular disease such as RAO and may replace more invasive conventional approaches that require administration of an intravenous dye.

OCTA is a useful diagnostic tool used to demonstrate the features necessary to diagnose RAO. Compared to FA, OCTA is fast, noninvasive, and can provide improved visualization of microvascular details. The features of disrupted flow in RAO are apparent with both dynamic FA and static OCTA imaging. Due to the nature of RAO, a static representation may be sufficient to make the diagnosis. OCTA can be used to accurately image retinal capillary networks at different levels in RAO and may be sufficiently sensitive to demonstrate the extent of ischemia in different vascular networks and to monitor vascular flow changes during the disease course.

PAMM lesions (i.e. INL infarcts) can be imaged accurately and noninvasively by OCTA and en face imaging, and recent studies have confirmed associated hypoperfusion and pathophysiological mechanisms behind DCP ischemia. Ischemia-reperfusion injury may be responsible for the pathogenesis and evolution of some PAMM lesions. While focal acute PAMM lesions may have preserved perfusion, old PAMM lesions develop a corresponding loss of flow and pruning within the DCP. Diffuse PAMM lesions occurring in the setting of CRAO lead to nonperfusion of the DCP in both acute and chronic instances.

References

[1] Leavitt JA, Larson TA, Hodge DO, Gullerud RE. The incidence of central retinal artery occlusion in Olmsted County, Minnesota. Am J Ophthalmol. 2011; 152(5):820–3.e2

[2] Hayreh SS. Acute retinal arterial occlusive disorders. Prog Retin Eye Res. 2011; 30(5):359–394

[3] Rahimy E, Kuehlewein L, Sadda SR, Sarraf D. Paracentral acute middle maculopathy: what we knew then and what we know now. Retina. 2015; 35(10):1921–1930

[4] Bonini Filho MA, Adhi M, de Carlo TE, et al. Optical coherence tomography angiography in retinal artery occlusion. Retina. 2015; 35(11):2339–2346

[5] Spaide RF, Klancnik JM, Jr, Cooney MJ. Retinal vascular layers imaged by fluorescein angiography and optical coherence tomography angiography. JAMA Ophthalmol. 2015; 133(1):45–50

[6] Damento G, Chen MH, Leng T. Spectral-domain optical cohe-rence tomography angiography of central retinal artery occlusion. Ophthalmic Surg Lasers Imaging Retina. 2016; 47(5):467–470

[7] Mastropasqua R, Di Antonio L, Di Staso S, et al. Optical coherence tomography angiography in retinal vascular diseases and choroidal neovascularization. J Ophthalmol. 2015; 2015:343515

[8] Shahlaee A, Samara WA, Sridhar J, et al. Accentuation of OCT angiography projection artifacts on hyperreflective retinal layers. Acta Ophthalmol (Copenh). 2016 Jul 1

[9] Chen X, Rahimy E, Sergott RC, et al. Spectrum of retinal vascular diseases associated with paracentral acute middle maculopathy. Am J Ophthalmol. 2015; 160(1):26–34.e1

[10] Sarraf D, Rahimy E, Fawzi AA, et al. Paracentral acute middle maculopathy: a new variant of acute macular neuroretinopathy associated with retinal capillary ischemia. JAMA Ophthalmol. 2013; 131(10):1275–1287

[11] Sridhar J, Shahlaee A, Rahimy E, et al. Optical coherence tomography angiography and en face optical coherence tomography features of paracentral acute middle maculopathy. Am J Ophthalmol. 2015; 160(6):1259–1268.e2

[12] Christenbury JG, Klufas MA, Sauer TC, Sarraf D. OCT angiography of paracentral acute middle maculopathy associated with central retinal artery occlusion and deep capillary ischemia. Ophthalmic Surg Lasers Imaging Retina. 2015; 46(5):579–581

[13] Khan MA, Rahimy E, Shahlaee A, Hsu J, Ho AC. En face optical coherence tomography imaging of deep capillary plexus abnormalities in paracentral acute middle maculopathy. Ophthalmic Surg Lasers Imaging Retina. 2015; 46(9):972–975

[14] Nemiroff J, Kuehlewein L, Rahimy E, et al. Assessing deep retinal capillary ischemia in paracentral acute middle maculopathy by optical coherence tomography angiography. Am J Ophthalmol. 2016; 162:121–132.e1

[15] Pecen PE, Smith AG, Ehlers JP. Optical coherence tomography angiography of acute macular neuroretinopathy and paracentral acute middle maculopathy. JAMA Ophthalmol. 2015; 133(12):1478–1480

[16] Casalino G, Williams M, McAvoy C, Bandello F, Chakravarthy U. Optical coherence tomography angiography in paracentral acute middle maculopathy secondary to central retinal vein occlusion. Eye (Lond). 2016; 30(6):888–893

[17] Shahlaee A, Samara WA, Hsu J, et al. in vivo assessment of macular vascular density in healthy human eyes using optical coherence tomography angiography. Am J Ophthalmol. 2016; 165:39–46

[18] Park JJ, Soetikno BT, Fawzi AA. Characterization of the middle capillary plexus using optical coherence tomography angiography in healthy and diabetic eyes. Retina. 2016; 36 (11):2039–2050

[19] de Carlo TE, Salz DA, Waheed NK, Baumal CR, Duker JS, Witkin AJ. Visualization of the retinal vasculature using wide-field montage optical coherence tomography angiography. Ophthalmic Surg Lasers Imaging Retina. 2015; 46(6):611–616

[20] Zhang Q, Lee CS, Chao J, et al. Wide-field optical coherence tomography based microangiography for retinal imaging. Sci Rep. 2016; 6:22017

[21] Zhang M, Hwang TS, Campbell JP, et al. Projection-resolved optical coherence tomographic angiography. Biomed Opt Express. 2016; 7(3):816–828

9 Optical Coherence Tomography Angiography in Retinal Venous Occlusions

Mostafa Hanout, Paulo Ricardo Chaves de Oliveira, and Alan R. Berger

Summary

Retinal venous occlusive disease (RVO) is characterized by vascular changes, which include dilation and engorgement of central or branch retinal veins, retinal hemorrhages, accumulation of intraretinal or subretinal fluid, and varying degrees of retinal ischemia. If the vascular changes affect the central macular area, RVO causes varying degrees of vision loss. Fundus fluorescein angiography has been the gold standard imaging technique to assess changes in retinal vasculature in RVO; however, it is an invasive technique and it lacks information about deeper vascular network. Optical coherence tomography (OCT) is a useful and widely popular imaging tool that provides high-resolution cross-sectional scans of the retina. OCT angiography (OCTA) has recently emerged as a novel noninvasive imaging modality that can generate a full map of the retinal vasculature that allows accurate evaluation of retinal vasculature in RVO. Recent studies have shown that OCTA is an excellent imaging modality to show vascular abnormalities associated with RVO including enlargement and disruption of the foveal avascular zone (FAZ), macular edema, microaneurysm formation, vascular looping, formation of venous–venous collaterals, capillary nonperfusion, and abnormal retinal neovascularization. Owing to its novelty, OCTA is not yet widely available in retina practices. Despite its limitations, such as small field of view, OCTA still offers numerous advantages over conventional fluorescein angiography. In addition, it is the first noninvasive imaging modality that can visualize the deep vascular network.

Keywords: optical coherence tomography, angiography, retinal vein occlusion, superficial vascular network, deep vascular network

9.1 Introduction

Retinal venous occlusive disease (RVO) is a vascular disorder that features dilation and engorgement of central or branch retinal veins, retinal hemorrhages, accumulation of intraretinal or subretinal fluid, and varying degrees of retinal ischemia. RVO is a very common cause of retinovascular vision loss, ranking second only to diabetic retinopathy.[1,2] Several population-based studies reported variable estimates of RVO prevalence that range from 0.3 to 2.3% in different ethnic groups.[3,4,5,6]

Significant vision loss in RVO typically occurs due to macular edema, macular ischemic changes, or as a sequela of complications related to retinal neovascularization. Fundus fluorescein angiography (FFA) is currently the gold standard imaging modality to assess retinal vasculature. FFA allows evaluation of vascular abnormalities in RVO such as retinal perfusion status, retinal neovascularization, delayed vascular filling, and intraretinal fluid leakage secondary to abnormal vascular permeability.[7,8] In the less severe nonischemic form of RVO, FFA shows staining along retinal veins, microaneurysms, dilated optic nerve head capillaries, and, occasionally, minimal areas of capillary nonperfusion. In the more severe ischemic form of RVO, FFA often shows marked hypofluorescence indicative of either capillary nonperfusion or blockage from diffuse retinal hemorrhages.[9] Intravenous fluorescein angiography, however, is invasive and involves intravenous injection of fluorescent chemical dye with the risk of associated adverse events such as nausea, vomiting, and, uncommonly, anaphylaxis. In addition, the detection and evaluation of deeper layers of retinal vasculature is not possible with FFA due to blockage by the fluorescence of the superficial vasculature.[7]

Optical coherence tomography (OCT) is a noninvasive imaging technique that provides high-resolution structural tomographic images of the multiple layers of the retina.[10] Optical coherence tomography angiography (OCTA) is a recent advance that compares the decorrelation (change) in the intensity of the OCT signal and/or phase variance of reflected light waves between successive cross-sectional B-scans to detect erythrocyte motion to construct high-resolution three-dimensional en face angiograms of chorioretinal vasculature. Generated angiograms can also be correlated with corresponding high-resolution OCT B-scans for better and more comprehensive assessment.[11] The authors have experience with the commercially available device Optovue XR Avanti with AngioVue software (Optovue, Fremont, CA). With this system, en face areas of 2 × 2, 3 × 3, 6 × 6, and

8×8 mm can be acquired. Since the same number of B-scans is acquired regardless of the scanned area, the larger the field of view, the lower the scan resolution. The 3×3 mm scans provide higher resolution compared to FFA without the risk of systemic complications.

9.2 Evaluation of the Fovea Avascular Zone

Physiologically, the fovea avascular zone (FAZ) is a capillary-free circular zone, approximately 450 to 600 µm in diameter at the center of the fovea surrounded by a ring of retinal capillaries.[12] In RVO, different morphological alterations take place in the FAZ especially in ischemic disease, which is characterized by disruption and enlargement of the FAZ ring. Enlargement of the FAZ indicates foveomacular ischemia.[13] Vessels close to the FAZ ring may also show vascular attenuation, tortuosity, looping, or microaneurysm formation ($\blacktriangleright$ Fig. 9.1a–e). The high resolution of OCTA scanning makes it more likely to detect FAZ changes and allows it to more clearly delineate microvascular malformations, which could be obscured by dye leakage on FFA.[14]

OCTA is the first imaging modality that enables noninvasive evaluation of the deep vascular plexus

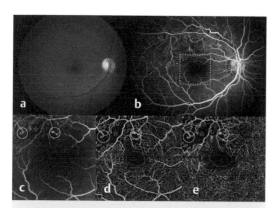

Fig. 9.1 Details of the foveal avascular zone (FAZ) in a 55-year-old female patient with a history of superotemporal branch retinal vein occlusion in her right eye for 18 months. **(a)** Color fundus photography. **(b)** Venous phase fluorescein angiography. **(c)** Magnified fluorescein angiography image of the yellow square in **(b)**; optical coherence tomography angiography at the level of the **(d)** superficial and **(e)** deep vascular networks showing enlargement of the FAZ (blue dashed line) and disruption of its normal contour. **(d)** and **(e)** also show nonperfused areas (red asterisks), vascular loops/tortuosity, and microaneurysms (yellow circles).

(DVP). There is a growing body of scientific evidence to support the belief that FAZ changes in RVO, especially disruption and enlargement of the FAZ ring, are often more pronounced at the level of the DVP.[15] This finding is obscured in FFA and can only be appreciated by OCTA. A recent clinical study showed statistically significant enlargement of FAZ maximum diameter measured by OCTA in eyes with RVO compared to normal healthy eyes ($p < 0.008$). Moreover, the same study showed strong correlation between best corrected visual acuity (BCVA) and FAZ maximum area measured by OCTA at the level of the DVP, hence highlighting the increasing importance of OCTA in evaluating the DVP ($\blacktriangleright$ Fig. 9.1c–e).[16]

9.3 Macular Edema

Macular edema is a common feature in RVO that may be present in both ischemic and non-ischemic forms of the disease. It represents the most common cause of vision loss in both branch and central RVO. The majority of patients with CRVO develop macular edema, whereas the incidence of macular edema is 5 to 15% in patients with BRVO.[17,18]

Conventional FFA demonstrates macular edema in the form of cystoid spaces or dye leakage in the mid to late phases of the angiogram. OCT, however, is more useful and more commonly used in quantifying and monitoring macular edema in patients with RVO, and is critical to the decision-making process in whether to treat or observe.[19] OCTA has the advantage of cross-registration of the en face scans of superficial vascular plexus (SVP) and DVP with the cross-sectional high-resolution OCT B-scans. Cystoid spaces of macular edema can be seen with OCT-A at the level of superficial or deep vascular networks as defined rounded or oblong areas with smooth borders that lack OCT signals and correspond well to the intraretinal cysts on OCT B-scan ($\blacktriangleright$ Fig. 9.2a–c).

9.4 Assessment of Retinal Perfusion and Vascular Abnormalities

Areas of capillary nonperfusion and microvascular changes such as telangiectatic vessels, microaneurysms, and venous–venous collaterals are commonly seen in RVO. Traditional FFA is a useful tool to characterize vascular abnormalities in RVO disease, such as delayed filling of the occluded retinal vein, capillary nonperfusion, microaneurysms,

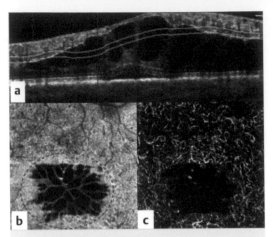

Fig. 9.2 Macular edema in a case of central retinal vein occlusion. **(a)** Cross-sectional optical coherence tomography (OCT) showing hyporeflective areas that represent intraretinal cysts. **(b)** OCT en face and **(c)** OCT angiography at the level of the deep vascular network showing lack of OCT signal in well-defined rounded or oblong areas with smooth borders corresponding to the intraretinal cysts (blue dashed circle).

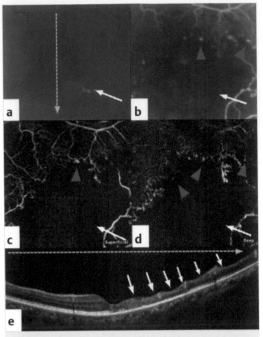

Fig. 9.3 Multimodal evaluation of a 63-year-old male patient, with a history of ischemic branch retinal vein occlusion in his left eye for 13 months. Visual acuity was 20/200. **(a)** Color fundus photography showing the presence of ghost vessels in the macular area (white arrow). The green dashed line indicates the position of the optical coherence tomography (OCT) cross-section shown in **(e)**. **(b)** Fluorescein angiography, OCT angiography of the **(c)** superficial plexus, and **(d)** deep plexus show the vessels are nonperfused (white arrow). Examples of microaneurysms are also demonstrated (blue arrowheads). **(e)** Atrophy of the neurosensory retina is observed on the cross-sectional OCT in the inferior macula (yellow arrows).

macular edema, or retinal neovascularization. However, blocked fluorescence from dense retinal hemorrhages and/or pooled fluorescein from diffuse dye leakage in macular edema may obscure microvascular details and make interpretation of FFA images more difficult. In addition, the deep vascular network cannot be visualized.[20] Recently published retrospective observational case series investigated the ability of OCTA to detect areas of retinal nonperfusion and microvascular changes compared to conventional FFA in patients with macular edema secondary to BRVO. These studies found OCTA to be superior to FFA in several aspects.[21] Out of 28 eyes included in the study, OCTA detected areas of nonperfusion in 28 eyes versus 18 eyes detected by FFA. Furthermore, the respective findings detected by OCTA and FFA were 13 and 11 eyes for superficial capillary telangiectasias, 28 and 11 eyes for deep capillary telangiectasias, 18 and 16 eyes for collateral vessels, and 13 and 14 eyes for microaneurysms (▶ Fig. 9.3a–e). Except for microaneurysms, OCTA appears to be more sensitive than FFA in detecting nonperfusion and all microvascular structural abnormalities. This is particularly evident in evaluating capillary nonperfusion and deep capillary telangiectasia. These findings can be explained by the fact that areas of nonperfusion may be more difficult to visualize in the presence of dye leakage, and inability of FFA to detect the deep capillary network, which

is believed to show more pronounced ischemia than superficial network. ▶ Fig. 9.3a–e demonstrates signs of retinal ischemia as detected by OCTA.

The Optovue OCT-A system (Optovue XR Avanti with AngioVue software) provides the option to automatically measure vascular density in the OCTA scan. The image can be divided into nine-sector grid, and vascular density can be measured in the whole scan and at each sector of the grid. Color-coded vascular density map can be generated with dark blue areas corresponding to areas of nonflow to facilitate detection of nonperfused regions (▶ Fig. 9.4).[22] Preretinal neovascularization may also be appreciated by OCTA, with fine details not obscured by leakage, as observed with conventional FFA (▶ Fig. 9.5).

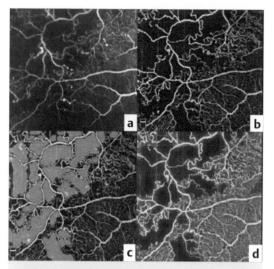

Fig. 9.4 Assessment of nonflow area and vessel density in a commercially available OCTA machine (Optovue XR Avanti with AngioVue software). Same patient as in ▶ Fig. 9.3. (a) Magnified fluorescein angiography of a localized area, superior to the macula. (b) A 3 × 3 mm OCT angiography at the level of the superficial vascular network. Vascular tortuosity, formation of collaterals, and areas of capillary nonperfusion can be appreciated. (c) Manual selection followed by automatic calculation of the capillary dropout/nonflow areas at the level of the superficial vascular network. (d) The vascular density is automatically calculated in the whole scan and in each grid pattern area. A color-coded map is provided where dark blue regions represent areas of nonflow.

9.5 Optic Nerve Head Evaluation

Optic nerve head abnormalities secondary to RVO can be detected by OCTA. Optociliary shunt vessels can be detected with sharp delineation by OCTA, whereas they can be blurred in color fundus photographs or FFA by flame-shaped retinal or disc hemorrhages (▶ Fig. 9.6). Similarly, neovascularization of the disc can be precisely appreciated by OCTA.

9.6 Conclusion

OCTA has shown several notable diagnostic advantages over conventional FFA for retinal vascular disorders such as RVO. The advantages include fast and noninvasive acquisition of images, lack of systemic adverse effects, automatic quantification of FAZ area, cross-registration with OCT B-scan, which enables structural, alongside vascular, evaluation, and above all its ability to evaluate deep vascular network. However, OCTA has not yet become established as a standard diagnostic method that is available in most retina practices. Novelty of the imaging technique and scant scientific clinical data may be partially responsible. The main limitations of OCTA, besides the small field of view and motion artifacts, include its inability to evaluate dynamic circulation and to display areas of vascular leakage. Continued development

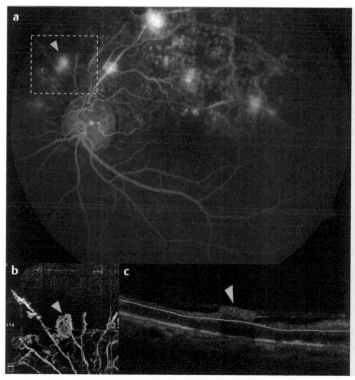

Fig. 9.5 A 69-year-old male patient with chronic branch retinal vein occlusion associated with preretinal neovascularization. (a) Multiple areas of leakage corresponding to preretinal neovascularization are observed in the fluorescein angiogram. (b) A 3 × 3 mm optical coherence tomography (OCT) angiogram of the corresponding yellow dashed square in (a) showing details of a preretinal neovascularization complex (green arrowhead) that was completely obscured by dye leakage in the fluorescein angiographic image. The co-registered OCT B scan (c) with angioverlay (red points demonstrate the presence of flow) delineating the segmentation boundaries of the OCT angiogram slab shown in (b), including the preretinal neovascular complex (green arrowhead) and superficial vascular network.

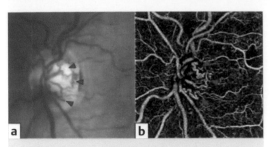

Fig. 9.6 A 51-year-old female patient with 13-month history of left central retinal vein occlusion and associated optociliary shunts. As observed in the **(a)** color fundus photograph, optical coherence tomography angiography of the **(b)** optic nerve head clearly delineates the optociliary shunts (blue arrowheads).

of the technique and further research that explores the limits of this technology and its optimum application are warranted.

References

[1] Ho M, Liu DT, Lam DS, Jonas JB. Retinal vein occlusions, from basics to the latest treatment. Retina. 2016; 36(3):432–448

[2] Woo SC, Lip GY, Lip PL. Associations of retinal artery occlusion and retinal vein occlusion to mortality, stroke, and myocardial infarction: a systematic review. Eye (Lond). 2016; 30(8):1031–1038

[3] Mitchell P, Smith W, Chang A. Prevalence and associations of retinal vein occlusion in Australia. The Blue Mountains Eye Study. Arch Ophthalmol. 1996; 114(10):1243–1247

[4] Klein R, Moss SE, Meuer SM, Klein BE. The 15-year cumulative incidence of retinal vein occlusion: the Beaver Dam Eye Study. Arch Ophthalmol. 2008; 126(4):513–518

[5] Klein R, Klein BE, Moss SE, Meuer SM. The epidemiology of retinal vein occlusion: the Beaver Dam Eye Study. Trans Am Ophthalmol Soc. 2000; 98:133–141, discussion 141–143

[6] Liu W, Xu L, Jonas JB. Vein occlusion in Chinese subjects. Ophthalmology. 2007; 114(9):1795–1796

[7] Spaide RF, Klancnik JM, Jr, Cooney MJ. Retinal vascular layers imaged by fluorescein angiography and optical coherence tomography angiography. JAMA Ophthalmol. 2015; 133(1): 45–50

[8] Rogers S, McIntosh RL, Cheung N, et al. International Eye Disease Consortium. The prevalence of retinal vein occlusion: pooled data from population studies from the United States, Europe, Asia, and Australia. Ophthalmology. 2010; 117(2): 313–9.e1

[9] The Central Vein Occlusion Study Group. Natural history and clinical management of central retinal vein occlusion. Arch Ophthalmol. 1997; 115(4):486–491

[10] Keane PA, Sadda SR. Retinal imaging in the twenty-first century: state of the art and future directions. Ophthalmology. 2014; 121(12):2489–2500

[11] Subhash HM, Leahy MJ. Microcirculation imaging based on full-range high-speed spectral domain correlation mapping optical coherence tomography. J Biomed Opt. 2014; 19(2): 21103

[12] Chui TY, Zhong Z, Song H, Burns SA. Foveal avascular zone and its relationship to foveal pit shape. Optom Vis Sci. 2012; 89(5):602–610

[13] Parodi MB, Visintin F, Della Rupe P, Ravalico G. Foveal avascular zone in macular branch retinal vein occlusion. Int Ophthalmol. 1995; 19(1):25–28

[14] Novais EA, Waheed NK. Optical coherence tomography angiography of retinal vein occlusion. Dev Ophthalmol. 2016; 56:132–138

[15] Coscas F, Glacet-Bernard A, Miere A, et al. Optical coherence tomography angiography in retinal vein occlusion: evaluation of superficial and deep capillary plexa. Am J Ophthalmol. 2016; 161:160–171.e1, 2

[16] Wons J, Pfau M, Wirth MA, Freiberg FJ, Becker MD, Michels S. Optical coherence tomography angiography of the foveal avascular zone in retinal vein occlusion. Ophthalmologica. 2016; 235(4):195–202

[17] McIntosh RL, Rogers SL, Lim L, et al. Natural history of central retinal vein occlusion: an evidence-based systematic review. Ophthalmology. 2010; 117(6):1113–1123.e15

[18] Rogers SL, McIntosh RL, Lim L, et al. Natural history of branch retinal vein occlusion: an evidence-based systematic review. Ophthalmology. 2010; 117(6):1094–1101.e5

[19] Lerche RC, Schaudig U, Scholz F, Walter A, Richard G. Structural changes of the retina in retinal vein occlusion: imaging and quantification with optical coherence tomography. Ophthalmic Surg Lasers. 2001; 32(4):272–280

[20] Mendis KR, Balaratnasingam C, Yu P, et al. Correlation of histologic and clinical images to determine the diagnostic value of fluorescein angiography for studying retinal capillary detail. Invest Ophthalmol Vis Sci. 2010; 51(11):5864–5869

[21] Suzuki N, Hirano Y, Yoshida M, et al. Microvascular abnormalities on optical coherence tomography angiography in macular edema associated with branch retinal vein occlusion. Am J Ophthalmol. 2016; 161:126–32.e1

[22] Samara WA, Shahlaee A, Sridhar J, Khan MA, Ho AC, Hsu J. Quantitative optical coherence tomography angiography features and visual function in eyes with branch retinal vein occlusion. Am J Ophthalmol. 2016; 166:76–83

10 Optical Coherence Tomography Angiography and Central Serous Chorioretinopathy

Wasim A. Samara, Carl D. Regillo, and Allen C. Ho

Summary

This chapter demonstrates the findings of optical coherence tomography angiography (OCTA) in the acute and chronic forms of central serous chorioretinopathy (CSC). CSC is a relatively common cause of vision loss and usually affects middle-aged males. Given that CSC disease activity is thought to reside in the choroidal vasculature, the ability to capture depth-resolved information about the retinal and choroidal circulation is of particular importance in this condition. OCTA appears to be a promising technology as it precludes the need of intravenous dye injection and provides depth-resolved three-dimensional information about the retinal and choroidal blood flow. Additionally, OCTA proves to be very useful in cases of chronic CSC associated with choroidal neovascularization (CNV) and can detect it in rates comparable to the invasive conventional imaging modalities. Given the noninvasive nature, OCTA could at least be considered as a first step in cases of CSC with suspected CNV and might even replace the need for fluorescein angiography in the near future. Nevertheless, interpretation of OCTA scans in CSC should be done with caution because the disrupted retinal anatomy might result in segmentation errors.

Keywords: acute central serous chorioretinopathy, chronic central serous chorioretinopathy, OCT angiography, optical coherence tomography, fluorescein angiography, indocyanine green angiography, choroidal neovascularization

10.1 Introduction

Central serous chorioretinopathy (CSC) is a disorder characterized by serous detachment of the neurosensory retina, sometimes accompanied by retinal pigment epithelium (RPE) detachment.[1,2] The serous detachment is caused by leakage of fluid through the RPE, which usually occurs at the macula, resulting in central vision loss.[1] Few risk factors have been associated with CSC including systemic corticosteroid use, type A personality, pregnancy, and endogenous Cushing's syndrome with most CSC cases occurring in young males.[2] While the pathophysiology is not fully understood,

different imaging modalities have shown that the subretinal fluid (SRF) accumulation in CSC results from hyperpermeability and congestion of the choroidal vasculature leading to SRF leakage through a dysfunctional RPE.[3]

Two forms of CSC can be distinguished: the acute and chronic variants.[1] Acute CSC usually presents with sudden visual loss and while spontaneous resolution is common with acute CSC, the chronic variant usually is progressive with persistence of the SRF for more than 3 months.[2,4] The acute form is characterized by focal leaks in the RPE that are clearly visible with fluorescein angiography (FA).[2,4] The chronic form is characterized by multifocal diffuse leakage evident with FA and indocyanine green angiography (ICGA), in addition to widespread RPE changes.[1] The persistent serous detachment in the chronic form results in progressive photoreceptor compromise, which explains the worse visual outcome with chronic CSC when compared to the acute form.[5] Chronic CSC might also be complicated with choroidal neovascularization (CNV).[1]

FA and ICGA have been the conventional imaging modalities to assess the vasculature in CSC. However, these tests remain invasive and time-consuming with potential side effects.[6] Recently, the development of optical coherence tomography angiography (OCTA) has allowed for three-dimensional visualization of the retinal and choroidal vasculature in a fast and noninvasive manner. This technology utilizes an algorithm called "split-spectrum amplitude decorrelation angiography," which is able to image the vasculature by using the contrast between the decorrelation of blood flow and static tissue to extract flow signals without requiring dye injection.[7] In this chapter, we describe the OCTA findings in eyes with CSC. Additionally, we briefly review the current literature on OCTA use in CSC. Of note, the OCTA scans represented in this chapter have been acquired using the commercially available RTvue XR Avanti spectral-domain OCT (SD-OCT) device with AngioVue software (Optovue, Inc., Fremont, CA).

10.2 Acute Central Serous Chorioretinopathy

In acute CSC, OCTA shows no flow abnormalities at the level of the superficial (SCP) and deep capillary

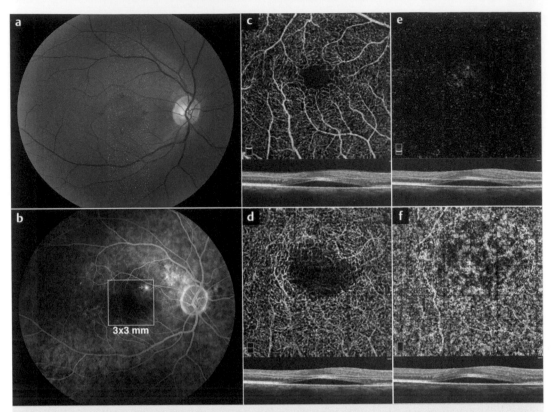

Fig. 10.1 Multimodal imaging of the right eye of a 48-year-old man complaining of blurry vision of 1-week duration, diagnosed with acute central serous chorioretinopathy. **(a)** Fundus image showing a shallow serous retinal detachment (SRD; arrows). **(b)** Late frame fluorescein angiogram showing a pinpoint leak in the macula (arrow). **(c–f)** optical coherence tomography angiography (OCTA) scans of 3 × 3 mm centered on the fovea (top) with co-registered B-scans showing the respective segmentation for each OCTA scan (bottom) taken using the AngioVue OCTA software on the commercially available RTvue XR Avanti device. **(c,d)** OCTA scans at the level of the **(c)** superficial and **(d)** deep capillary plexus with a normal flow pattern. **(e)** OCTA scan at the level of the outer retina shows trace flow as a result of projection artifacts from the superficial and deep capillary flow. **(f)** OCTA at the level of the choriocapillaris demonstrating an area of increased choroidal flow among a dark area (yellow trace) that corresponds to the overlying SRD.

plexus (DCP; ▶ Fig. 10.1). However, before interpreting OCTA scans in any case of CSC, it is crucial to recognize that due to the detachment of the neurosensory retina, segmentation errors can arise and affect the scan interpretation. One should make sure that the segmentation lines on the co-registered B-scans correspond to the correct retinal layers before reading the scans. When flow abnormalities are seen in SCP or DCP, these can be explained by the aforementioned segmentation errors. After correcting the segmentation, normal flow patterns can be seen.

At the level of the choriocapillaris (30–60 μ below the RPE), OCTA shows flow abnormalities. First, areas of increased choroidal flow can be seen

under the area of serous retinal detachment (SRD) representing an area of disease activity (▶ Fig. 10.1). Second, a dark area of an apparent flow reduction can be noticed corresponding to the area of the SRD. We hypothesize that this area is not a true reduction in choroidal flow but rather an artifact due to light attenuation by the overlying SRD. Alternatively, compression of the choriocapillaris by the enlarged vessels in the outer choroid can lead to focal atrophy with an actual reduction in blood flow[8] and could explain this finding.

Recent studies have used OCTA to describe vascular changes in acute CSC. Feucht and colleagues have similarly shown that there were no vascular abnormalities seen at the level of SCP and DCP. At the choriocapillaris level, irregular blood flow patterns were described with areas of hypoperfusion surrounded by areas of hyperperfusion.[9] Another study also found that the choriocapillaris shows an area of apparent flow reduction surrounded by an area of increased flow.[10]

It is important to note that the previously described OCTA changes at the level of the choriocapillaris are nonspecific given the inability of the current spectral domain OCTA devices to image the choroid accurately. This is partially due to the high reflectivity of the RPE limiting the penetration of the light beam into the choroid. Additionally, the current devices use short wavelengths, which also limit the penetration into the choroid. However, the development of swept-source OCTA utilizing higher wavelengths will allow increased light penetration and improved choroidal blood flow visualization compared to the light source used in the currently available SD-OCT devices.

10.3 Chronic Central Serous Chorioretinopathy

In chronic CSC, OCTA reveals normal retinal circulation (SCP and DCP) similar to the acute form. At the choroidal level, OCTA shows irregular flow patterns that correspond with abnormalities seen on ICGA (▶ Fig. 10.2). The choriocapillaris shows areas of hypoperfusion surrounded by areas of hyperperfusion. Earlier studies have demonstrated focal filling defects in the choriocapillaris with dilated arterioles and venules.[3] These

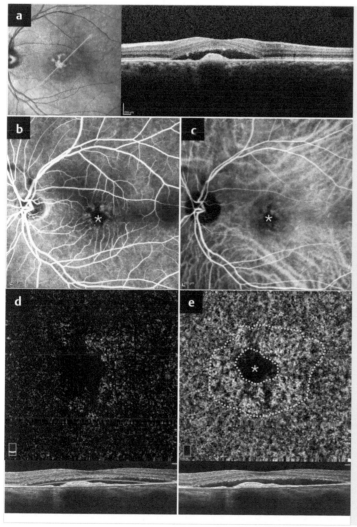

Fig. 10.2 Multimodal imaging of the left eye of a 59-year-old woman with chronic central serous chorioretinopathy previously treated with photodynamic therapy. (a) Radial spectral-domain optical coherence tomography (SD-OCT) scan showing serous retinal detachment and a heterogeneously hyper-reflective retinal pigment epithelium detachment (RPED; asterisk). (b) Late frame fluorescein angiogram showing multiple leakage points surrounding an area of dye blockage (asterisk) secondary to the RPED. (c) Late frame indocyanine green angiography showing abnormal dilation of the choroidal vessels with an area of dye blockage (asterisk) secondary to the RPED. (d,e) OCT angiography (OCTA) scans of 3 × 3 mm centered on the fovea (top) with co-registered B-scans showing the respective segmentation for each OCTA scan (bottom) taken using the AngioVue OCTA software on the commercially available RTvue XR Avanti device. (d) A 3 × 3 mm OCTA scan at the level of the outer retina showing absence of flow with shadowing artifact in the area corresponding to the RPED (asterisk), excluding the possibility of an associated choroidal neovascularization. (e) OCTA scan at the level of the choriocapillaris demonstrating shadowing artifact secondary to the RPED (asterisk) surrounded by an area of increased choroidal flow (yellow trace).

choriocapillary changes seem to persist even after the resolution of the SRF.

The diagnosis of CNV associated with chronic CSC can be often challenging as many clinical features are shared between CSC with and without CNV. These changes include RPE detachment, intraretinal or SRF, retinal atrophy, and diffuse irregular hyperfluorescence seen on FA or ICGA.[11] OCTA is useful in these cases especially when the RPE profile is irregular with associated RPE detachments to rule out possible CNV (▶ Fig. 10.2). OCTA has recently been shown to be sensitive and specific for the detection of CNV in different disease entities. Of note, for the scans provided in this chapter, the outer retina automatic segmentation lines were manually adjusted where the inner boundary was set to be located at the outer boundary of the outer plexiform layer and the outer

boundary was set at the level of Bruch's membrane as previously described.[11] This has been shown to increase the sensitivity of OCTA to detect associated CNV.[11] In healthy eyes, the outer retina does not have any vascular structures; therefore, OCTA is not expected to show flow signal at the outer retina level, which makes identification of CNV lesions easier at this level.

The CNV associated with CSC shows different morphologies with either well-circumscribed (sea-fan-shaped vessels) or poorly circumscribed pattern (▶ Fig. 10.3 and ▶ Fig. 10.4). On follow-up after treatment with anti–vascular endothelial growth factor (anti-VEGF), OCTA demonstrates a decrease in the CNV size as well as decreased anastomosis in the vascular lesion, making it very useful in the longitudinal follow-up after treatment (▶ Fig. 10.4). In addition, latest OCTA software

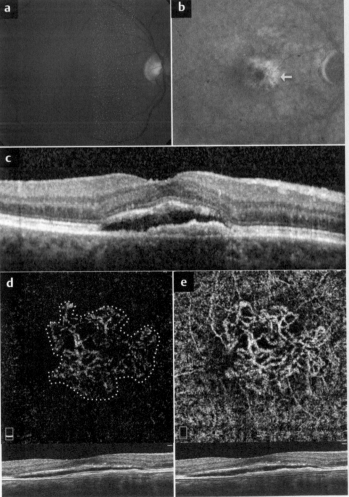

Fig. 10.3 Multimodal imaging of the right eye of a 68-year-old man with chronic central serous chorioretinopathy complicated by a type 1 choroidal neovascularization (CNV). **(a)** Fundus photograph showing chronic retinal pigment epithelium changes in the macula. **(b)** Late frame fluorescein angiogram showing the CNV as an area of subretinal dye leakage (arrow). **(c)** Horizontal spectral domain optical coherence tomography (OCT) scan through the fovea showing serous retinal detachment with an irregular retinal pigment epithelium detachment. **(d,e)** OCT angiography (OCTA) scans of 3 × 3 mm centered on the fovea (top) with co-registered B-scans showing the respective segmentation for each OCTA scan (bottom) taken using the AngioVue OCTA software on the commercially available RTvue XR Avanti device. **(d)** A 3 × 3 mm OCTA scan set at the level of the outer retina showing the presence of a distinct vascular network representing a CNV (yellow trace). **(e)** The CNV could also be seen on the OCTA scan taken at the choriocapillaris level.

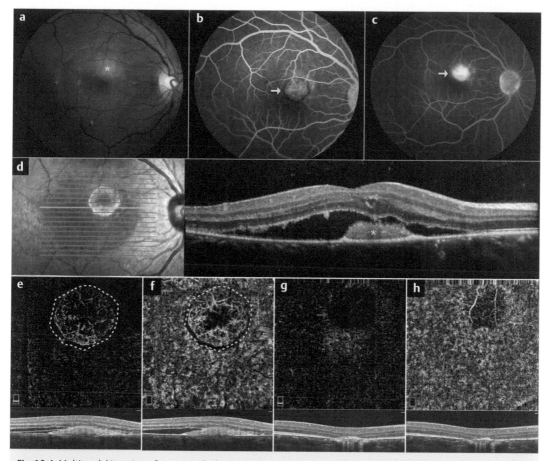

Fig. 10.4 Multimodal imaging of an eye with chronic central serous chorioretinopathy complicated by a type 2 choroidal neovascularization (CNV) in a 22-year-old man with a history of chronic use of topical steroid cream. **(a)** Fundus image showing serous retinal detachment (SRD; arrows) with an associated subretinal lesion (asterisk). **(b)** Early frame fluorescein angiogram (FA) showing the CNV as an area of subretinal hyperfluorescence (arrow). **(c)** On late-frame FA, the area of hyperfluorescence seen on early frames shows intense dye leakage (arrow). **(d)** Horizontal spectral-domain optical coherence tomography scan showing SRD and a type 2 CNV (asterisk). **(e–h)** OCT angiography (OCTA) scans of 3 × 3 mm centered on the fovea (top) with co-registered B-scans showing the respective segmentation for each OCTA scan (bottom) taken using the AngioVue OCTA software on the commercially available RTvue XR Avanti device. **(e–f)** OCTA at the level of the outer retina **(e)** and choriocapillaris **(f)** show a distinct vascular network representing a CNV (yellow trace). **(g,h)** On follow-up after treatment with intravitreal anti–vascular endothelial growth factor (anti-VEGF) injections, repeat scans at the level of the **(g)** outer retina and **(h)** choriocapillaris showed decreased size and reduction of flow within the CNV (arrows).

updates allow accurate measurement of the CNV size.

A recent study has demonstrated that OCTA is superior to other imaging modalities to detect CNV in chronic CSC cases. The authors demonstrated CNV in in 7 out of 12 study eyes (58%). Interestingly, these CNV lesions corresponded to the areas of hyperpermeability on ICGA. Moreover, the CNV lesions corresponded to the small undulating RPE detachments on B-scans.[12] The CNV lesions in that study could only be detected with OCTA and were not easily detected with FA or ICGA.[12] Another study looked at the sensitivity of OCTA in detecting CNV in chronic CSC. The investigators were able to detect all the CNV lesions detected by FA yielding 100% sensitivity.[11]

References

[1] Wang M, Munch IC, Hasler PW, Prünte C, Larsen M. Central serous chorioretinopathy. Acta Ophthalmol. 2008; 86(2):126–145

[2] Liew G, Quin G, Gillies M, Fraser-Bell S. Central serous chorioretinopathy: a review of epidemiology and pathophysiology. Clin Experiment Ophthalmol. 2013; 41(2):201–214

[3] Prünte C, Flammer J. Choroidal capillary and venous congestion in central serous chorioretinopathy. Am J Ophthalmol. 1996; 121(1):26–34

[4] Gemenetzi M, De Salvo G, Lotery AJ. Central serous chorioretinopathy: an update on pathogenesis and treatment. Eye (Lond). 2010; 24(12):1743–1756

[5] Loo RH, Scott IU, Flynn HW, Jr, et al. Factors associated with reduced visual acuity during long-term follow-up of patients with idiopathic central serous chorioretinopathy. Retina. 2002; 22(1):19–24

[6] Yannuzzi LA, Rohrer KT, Tindel LJ, et al. Fluorescein angiography complication survey. Ophthalmology. 1986; 93 (5):611–617

[7] Jia Y, Tan O, Tokayer J, et al. Split-spectrum amplitude-decorrelation angiography with optical coherence tomography. Opt Express. 2012; 20(4):4710–4725

[8] Yang L, Jonas JB, Wei W. Optical coherence tomography-assisted enhanced depth imaging of central serous chorioretinopathy. Invest Ophthalmol Vis Sci. 2013; 54(7): 4659–4665

[9] Feucht N, Maier M, Lohmann CP, Reznicek L. OCT angiography findings in acute central serous chorioretinopathy. Ophthalmic Surg Lasers Imaging Retina. 2016; 47(4):322–327

[10] Costanzo E, Cohen SY, Miere A, et al. Optical coherence tomography angiography in central serous chorioretinopathy. J Ophthalmol. 2015; 2015:134783

[11] -Bonini Filho MA, de Carlo TE, Ferrara D, et al. Association of choroidal neovascularization and central serous chorioretinopathy with optical coherence tomography angiography. JAMA Ophthalmol. 2015; 133(8):899–906

[12] Quaranta-El Maftouhi M, El Maftouhi A, Eandi CM. Chronic central serous chorioretinopathy imaged by optical coherence tomographic angiography. Am J Ophthalmol. 2015; 160(3): 581–587.e1

11 Optical Coherence Tomography Angiography in Macular Telangiectasia Type 2

Alain Gaudric and Valérie Krivosic

Summary

In macular telangiectasia type 2 (MacTel2), optical coherence tomography angiography (OCTA) shows capillary dilation and rarefaction in both the superficial capillary plexus and the deep capillary plexus (DCP), with a decreased density compared to normal. The anomaly is more pronounced on the temporal side of the fovea but may extend to the whole MacTel2 area, especially in the DCP. During the course of the disease, newly formed capillaries invade the outer nuclear layer in front of the areas of ellipsoid zone loss. This often corresponds to the development of a dilated right angle venule that drains the DCP and the outer intraretinal new vessels. At this stage, the foveal avascular zone is dragged temporally toward the emergence of the venule often embedded in a fibrotic and pigmented tissue. At more advanced stages, OCTA shows the network of subretinal vessels on the retinal pigment epithelium (RPE) surface contained in a fibrous and pigmented plaque and elevating the retina from the RPE.

Keywords: macular telangiectasia type 2, MacTel2, optical coherence tomography angiography, subretinal new vessels, intraretinal new vessels, ellipsoid zone

11.1 Introduction

Macular telangiectasia type 2 (MacTel2) is a progressive neurogliovascular macular dystrophy starting in the fifth decade of life and evolving progressively toward macular atrophy.[1]

When the disease becomes symptomatic, some capillary changes are already present and are characterized by "occult" telangiectasia, mainly on the temporal side of the macula, and often, but not always, associated with a slightly dilated venule originating at right angle from the temporal side of the macula.

Telangiectasia is associated with structural retinal changes such as loss of macular pigment, whitening of the inner retina, crystal deposition in the optic nerve fiber layer, cystic formation in the inner part of the fovea, and outer cavitation. Lastly in some advanced stages of the disease, subretinal

new vessels may proliferate from the deep capillary plexus (DCP) and result in bleeding or fibrosis beneath the retina.[1]

MacTel2 is well imaged by conventional multimodal imaging.[2] Fundus autofluorescence (FAF) shows early changes in macular pigment density,[3] blue reflectance photograph shows the whitening of the inner retina as a temporal crescent or an oval area occupying the whole macula,[4] fluorescein angiography (FA) shows a mild leakage and staining of the retinal tissue at the telangiectasia but no filling of the cystic macular spaces, and structural optical coherence tomography (OCT) shows the inner macular cysts and outer cavitations. En face OCT also shows the areas of ellipsoid zone (EZ) breakdown in the vicinity of the foveal center, as well as microcavitations[5] in the inner nuclear layer and ganglion cell layer, extending through the whole area of the "MacTel" zone. Finally, adaptive optics (AO) has shown the loss of photoreceptor cells in the areas of EZ breakdown, but with the persistence of some cone elements.[6,7]

OCT angiography (OCTA) provides new details of the telangiectasia, which gave their name to the disease, although they are only part of the disease spectrum.

Before the era of OCT and modern multimodal imaging, Mactel2 (initially called idiopathic juxtafoveal telangiectasia[8]) were classified into five stages, which do not fit well with the anomalies observed nowadays. We will therefore use the terms "early," "intermediate," "advanced," and "atrophic" to describe the progressive increase in capillary anomaly severity, although another system of grading has been proposed recently based on OCTA.[9]

11.2 Early Stage with Isolated Telangiectasia

At an early stage, telangiectasias are barely visible on fundus examination, and only a minimal leakage is seen on FA. OCTA shows a mild dilation of both the superficial capillary plexus (SCP) and the DCP on the temporal side of the fovea. The capillary density ranges within normal values in both the SCP and the DCP. A venule draining the temporal part of the fovea may be slightly dilated (▶ Fig. 11.1).

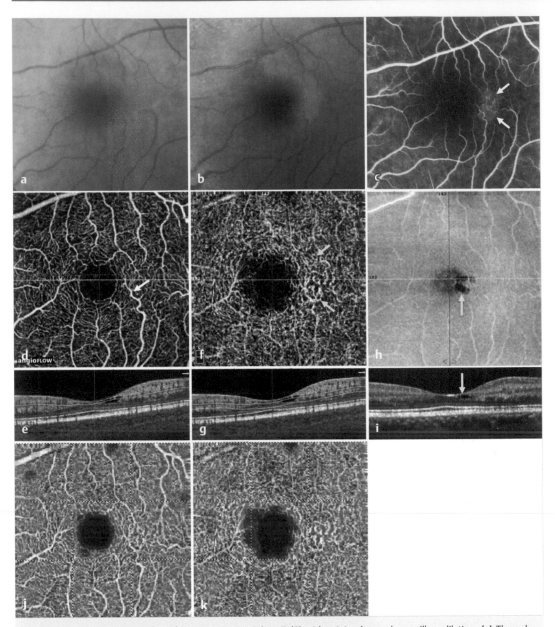

Fig. 11.1 Early stage of macular telangiectasia type 2 (MacTel2) with minimal macular capillary dilation. **(a)** The color photo shows no significant changes in the macula. **(b)** The blue reflectance image shows a temporomacular crescent of inner retinal whitening characteristic of the disease. **(c)** On fluorescein angiography, a mild hyperfluorescence is visible on the temporal side of the fovea (arrows) without clear visibility of telangiectasia. **(d)** Optical coherence tomography (OCT) angiogram segmented at the superficial capillary plexus (SCP) showing a very mild dilation of the superficial capillaries and a slightly tortuous venule (arrow). **(e)** Corresponding OCT B-scan showing only a small inner cystic cavity on the temporal side of the fovea. **(f)** Deep capillary plexus (DCP) with small dilated capillaries temporal to the fovea (arrows). **(g)** Corresponding OCT B-scan on which the vascular flow (red points) does not appear abnormal. **(h)** En face (nonflow) image showing the parafoveal inner cysts (arrow) with its correspondence on the **(i)** structural B-scan. Capillary density **(j)** at the SCP and **(k)** at the DCP ranging within normal values.

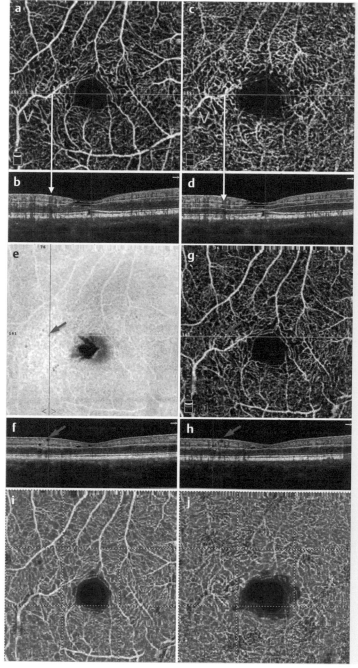

Fig. 11.2 Early stage of macular telangiectasia type 2 (MacTel2) with macular capillary and venular dilation. **(a)** Optical coherence tomography (OCT) angiogram segmented at the superficial capillary plexus (SCP) showing some degree of dilation of the superficial capillaries and an enlargement of the intercapillary space. A temporal venule (V) is slightly dilated (arrow) and corresponds on **(b)** the OCT B-scan to an increase in vascular flow. Note also the small cystic cavity in the temporal side of the fovea. **(c)** Deep capillary plexus (DCP) with more pronounced dilation of the deep capillaries and dilation of the deep part of the dilated venule (V), which corresponds on **(d)** the OCT B-scan to an increase in vascular flow (arrow). **(e,f)** En face (nonflow) image segmented at the SCP and corresponding OCT B-scan showing several microcysts (one of them marked by an arrow) located at various levels of the inner retina. Note also the stellate pattern of the inner foveal cysts in the temporal part of the fovea. **(g,h)** On the OCT angiogram of the DCP and on the corresponding OCT B-scan, these microcysts correspond to small capillary voids (arrows). **(i)** Capillary density at the SCP and **(j)** at the DCP are smaller than normal.

In other cases, a capillary dilation and an irregular pattern are more visible and more extended, especially in the DCP (▶ Fig. 11.2), and are associated with some capillary ectasia and a dilated draining venule. On the en face image, large cystic cavities are present on the temporal part of the foveal center, as well as other microcysts in the ganglion cell layer and inner nuclear layer, which correspond to small lacunae in the SCP and DCP. There is globally some degree of capillary rarefaction, mainly in the DCP, and a decrease in capillary density.[3,9,10]

11.3 Intermediate Stage with Outer Intraretinal New Vessels

At an intermediate stage, a dilated venule emerges on the temporal side of the macula and drains the cluster of coarse capillaries in the SCP and DCP, usually adjacent to inner foveal cystic spaces (▶ Fig. 11.3). The foveal avascular zone (FAZ) is dragged temporally,[5] and the capillaries of the SCP are rarefied and dilated. These capillary anomalies

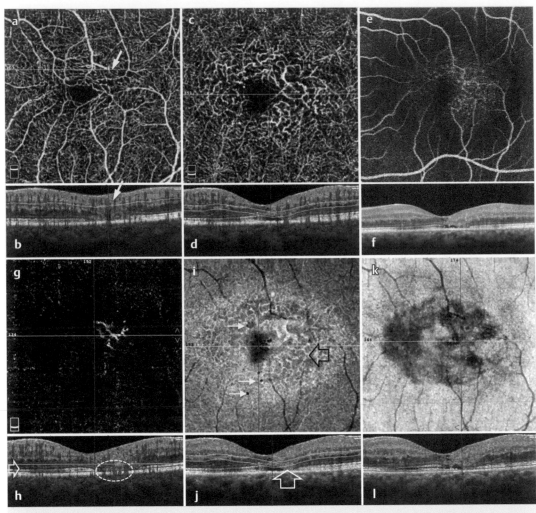

Fig. 11.3 Intermediate stage of macular telangiectasia type 2 (MacTel2) with outer intraretinal new vessels. **(a)** Optical coherence tomography (OCT) angiogram of the superficial capillary plexus (SCP) showing a dilated venule originating at right angle from the temporal part of the fovea (arrow). The capillaries are dilated and rarefied with increased intervascular spaces. The foveal avascular zone (FAZ) is slightly dragged temporally. **(b)** Corresponding OCT B-scan passing through the termination of the right angle venule showing an increased vascular flow at this level (arrow). **(c,d)** Coarse capillaries in the deep capillary plexus (DCP) and corresponding OCT B-scan. **(e,f)** Fluorescein angiography showing the dilated capillaries less distinctly than OCT angiography, and corresponding structural OCT B-scan. **(g,h)** Segmentation at the outer retina (large arrow) showing an abnormal capillary network in yellow **(g)** corresponding to the vascular flow just above the retinal pigment epithelium (ellipse) on **(h)** the OCT B-scan. **(i)** En face OCT (nonflow) segmented at the DCP. Note the presence of numerous microcysts (light arrows on some of them), and the visibility of some dilated coarse capillaries (large arrow). **(j)** Corresponding structural OCT B-scan showing the collapse of the outer nuclear layer on the retinal pigment epithelium (large arrow). **(k)** En face OCT segmented at the ellipsoid zone (EZ); the black area corresponds to the EZ loss. **(l)** Corresponding OCT B-scan with a double red line showing the segmentation at the EZ.

are more pronounced in the DCP where they extend to the whole macular area. Telangiectasia are better seen on OCTA than on FA.[9,11] Moreover, OCTA shows a subjacent layer of capillaries invading the outer nuclear layer (ONL) in front of the area of EZ loss temporal to the fovea.

A dilated venule and FAZ distortion may be associated with intraretinal pigment proliferation (► Fig. 11.4). These pigmentary plaques are well visible on color photos. On structural OCT, they appear as a hyper-reflective structure occupying almost the whole retinal thickness on the temporal side of the FAZ, in an area of EZ loss. On the OCT B-scan, their flow is relatively high and they are located at the convergence of telangiectatic capillaries into the right angle venule.[12]

Apart from the dilated DCP, an additional layer of newly formed capillaries invades the ONL. This is not a segmentation artifact due to the collapse of the ONL on the retinal pigment epithelium (RPE) but a true additional capillary network that does not have the same pattern as the DCP.[9,12,13,14,15] It is remarkable that these outer intraretinal new vessels occur in front of the area of EZ loss.[16]

11.4 Advanced Stage with Subretinal New Vessels and Fibrosis

Subretinal new vessels are suspected in the presence of subretinal fibrosis on the temporal side of the fovea associated with a pigmented plaque and dilated venule. A subretinal hemorrhage may also be associated. FA may show the contour of the neovascular membrane. On structural OCT, the subretinal vessels are embedded in a fibrous plaque, which appears hyper-reflective (► Fig. 11.5). The overlying retina is elevated and more or less edematous. The right angle venule draining the telangiectatic capillaries and subretinal new vessels corresponds to the vascular flow on the corresponding OCT B-scan. A large network of subretinal new vessels is surrounded by a hyper-reflective tissue containing the intraretinal pigment.[17] The presence of retinochoroidal anastomoses has been suggested in some publications,[11,15] but in general there is not enough evidence of such a connection between subretinal new vessels and the choroid.

11.5 Late Atrophic Stage

At an atrophic stage, the macula is abnormally thin due to the enlargement of the intraretinal cysts and ultimately to a collapse of the empty spaces. The capillary density decreases, but telangiectasias persist, including outer intraretinal new vessels persisting in a highly atrophic neuroglial tissue (► Fig. 11.6).

11.6 Conclusion

In MacTel2, the fact that telangiectasia appear secondarily to a neuroglial dysfunction is not definitively established, but there are some indications that specific morphological alterations precede vascular alterations and functional deficits, including an asymmetry of the foveal pit, and reduced optical density of the macular pigment in the temporal part of the fovea.[18] However as noted by Gillies,[19] parallel neuronal and vascular pathogenic pathways secondary to Müller cell dysfunction, whose cause remains obscure, may explain the course of MacTel2. In the earliest cases, we have been able to image with OCTA the capillary dilation that was minimal and the capillary density ranged within normal values in both the SCP and DCP. However, in all the other cases, the temporofoveal capillaries were dilated, irregular, with an enlargement of the intervascular space and a decrease in their density, and these findings were more pronounced in the DCP than in the SCP. The dilated temporofoveal venule(s) become visible mainly when (but sometimes before) newly formed capillaries proliferate in the normally avascular outer retina.[5] The FAZ is dragged to its temporal side toward the emergence of the dilated venule(s). In more advanced cases, the capillary changes are extended to the whole macular area.

The reason why, in Mactel2 disease, intraretinal new vessels may proliferate in the normally avascular ONL remains unclear. It is admitted that the progressive focal loss of photoreceptors is probably secondary to Müller cell dysfunction and death.[1,20] The impairment of the photoreceptors appears as a breakdown of the EZ and external limiting membrane (ELM), although cone inner segments have been histologically found in the areas of EZ loss. However, while some cones survive, there was a massive loss of rods.[20] Furthermore, we have shown that even in the absence of obvious EZ breakdown, the fragmentation of the interdigitation zone was related to a decrease in cone density on AO.[6] Another AO study has shown that cones may be abnormal and non–wave guiding despite the apparently normal reflectivity of the EZ in the parafovea.[21] It seems then paradoxical that a loss of photoreceptors, which are important oxygen

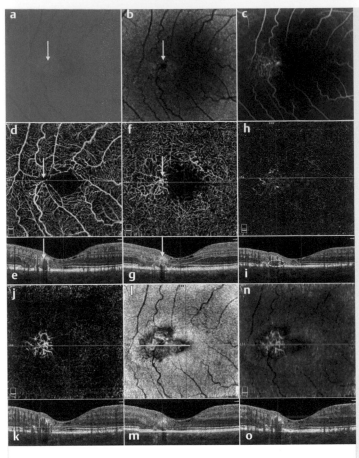

Fig. 11.4 Intermediate stage of macular telangiectasia type 2 (MacTel2) with outer intraretinal new vessels and intraretinal pigment proliferation. **(a)** Color photo showing a pigmented plaque temporal to the fovea (arrow) better seen on **(b)** the red-free filter image where it surrounds the extremity of a dilated venule (arrow). **(c)** Fluorescein angiography shows the capillary dilation on the temporal side of the fovea. **(d)** Superficial capillary plexus (SCP) with telangiectasia drained by a dilated venule (arrow). The foveal avascular zone (FAZ) is enlarged and dragged toward the pigmented plaque and dilated venule. **(e)** Corresponding optical coherence tomography (OCT) B-scan showing a high flow below the emergence of the dilated venule in the deeper part of the retina (arrow). **(f)** Deep capillary plexus (DCP) showing coarse capillaries converging toward the origin of the dilated venule, temporal to the fovea (arrow). **(g)** The structural OCT B-scan shows the increased focal reflectivity of the retinal tissue (arrow) underlying the extremity of the dilated venule and containing the vascular flow as seen in **(e)**. **(h)** OCT angiogram segmented at the posterior edge of the inner nuclear layer showing the deepest capillaries of the DCP (in purple) behind which an additional network is visible (in yellow). **(i)** Corresponding OCT B-scan at a level different from that of **(e)** showing the flow (ellipse) just above the retinal pigment epithelium (RPE). **(j)** OCT angiogram segmented above the RPE showing the network of outer intraretinal new vessels corresponding to the flow (red dots) seen in **(k)** above the RPE. **(l)** En face OCT segmented at the ellipsoid zone (EZ) showing a black area corresponding to the irregular patchy loss of EZ. The green line corresponds to the EZ loss seen on the structural OCT B-scan in **(m)**. **(n)** Superimposition of the outer intraretinal neovascular network on the en face image segmented at the EZ, showing that the intraretinal new vessels have proliferated in front of the area of EZ loss. **(o)** Corresponding abnormal flow on the OCT-A B-scan.

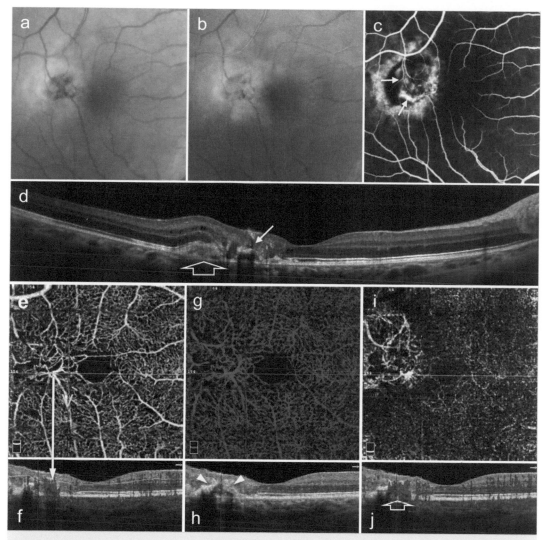

Fig. 11.5 Advanced stage of macular telangiectasia type 2 (Mactel2) with subretinal new vessels and fibrosis. **(a)** Color photo showing a subretinal whitish fibrous plaque and intraretinal pigment temporal to the fovea. **(b)** The blue reflectance image also shows the whitening of the whole macular area. **(c)** Fluorescein angiography showing the characteristic appearance of a subretinal neovascular membrane (arrows). **(d)** The optical coherence tomography (OCT) B-scan shows a subretinal hyper-reflective structure temporal to the fovea (large arrow) with some cystoid changes in the underlying retina. There is also some hyper-reflectivity from the intraretinal pigment proliferation (small arrow). **(e)** OCT angiogram at the superficial capillary plexus showing coarse capillaries drained by a dilated venule (V), corresponding to a high flow (arrow) on **(f)** the corresponding OCT B-scan. **(g)** OCT angiogram at the deep capillary plexus surrounded on the corresponding structural OCT B-scan **(h)** by a hyper-reflective intraretinal pigmentation (arrows). **(i)** OCT angiogram segmented above the retinal pigment epithelium showing the network of subretinal new vessels corresponding to the flow (large arrow) seen in **(j)**.

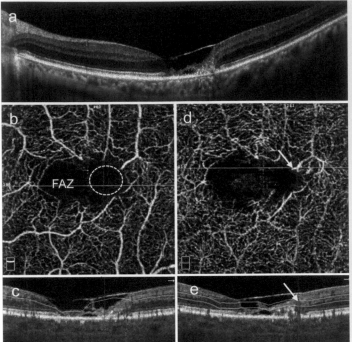

Fig. 11.6 Late atrophic stage of macular telangiectasia type 2 (MacTel2). **(a)** Horizontal optical coherence tomography (OCT) B-scan showing a large central cystic cavity with a partially open roof and a profound loss of retinal tissue. **(b)** OCT angiogram of the superficial capillary plexus showing an enlargement of the foveal avascular zone (FAZ) adjacent to an area of capillary void (ellipse) that corresponds to the portion of the cystic space seen on **(c)** the corresponding OCT B-scan. **(d)** OCT angiogram of the deep capillary plexus showing the abrupt emergence of a dilated venule at the edge of the cystic space (arrow), which corresponds on **(e)** the OCT B-scan to a flow signal in the outer retina (arrow). There is overall a rarefaction of the retinal capillaries in the MacTel area.

consumers, may lead to a proliferation of the retinal capillary toward the RPE because it is likely that there is no hypoxia stimulus under these conditions.

However, several animal models resulting in photoreceptor impairment have also led to the abnormal vascularization of the outer retina,[22,23,24,25] and especially in areas of photoreceptor loss or degeneration.[22,24] Moreover, a transgenic mouse model resulting in a selective ablation of Muller cells leading to photoreceptor apoptosis has also resulted in the growth of deep retinal new vessels.[26] The fact that, in our patients, the deep retinal capillaries invaded the outer retina specifically in the area of EZ loss, which is considered a marker of photoreceptor impairment, fits well with this transgenic mouse model with dysfunctional Müller cells. It is thus likely that a mechanism other than hypoxia promotes the outer capillary proliferation in Mactel2 eyes, including the loss of anti-angiogenic factors normally produced by the photoreceptors and Muller cells.[5,16]

11.7 Disclosure

Dr. A. Gaudric and V. Krivosic participate to the International MacTel Project (http://www.mactel-research.org).

References

[1] Charbel Issa P, Gillies MC, Chew EY, et al. Macular telangiectasia type 2. Prog Retin Eye Res. 2013; 34:49–77

[2] Sallo FB, Leung I, Clemons TE, et al. Multimodal imaging in type 2 idiopathic macular telangiectasia. Retina. 2015; 35(4): 742–749

[3] Zeimer M, Gutfleisch M, Heimes B, Spital G, Lommatzsch A, Pauleikhoff D. Association between Changes in macular vasculature in optical coherence tomography- and fluorescein-angiography and distribution of macular pigment in type 2 idiopathic macular telangiectasia. Retina. 2015; 35(11):2307–2316

[4] Charbel Issa P, Berendschot TT, Staurenghi G, Holz FG, Scholl HP. Confocal blue reflectance imaging in type 2 idiopathic macular telangiectasia. Invest Ophthalmol Vis Sci. 2008; 49 (3):1172–1177

[5] Spaide RF, Suzuki M, Yannuzzi LA, Matet A, Behar-Cohen F. Volume-rendered angiographic and structural optical coherence tomography angiography of macular telangiectasia type 2. Retina. 2017; 37(3):424–435

[6] Jacob J, Krivosic V, Paques M, Tadayoni R, Gaudric A. Cone density loss on adaptive optics in early macular telangiectasia type 2. Retina. 2016; 36(3):545–551

[7] Wang Q, Tuten WS, Lujan BJ, et al. Adaptive optics microperimetry and OCT images show preserved function and recovery of cone visibility in macular telangiectasia type 2 retinal lesions. Invest Ophthalmol Vis Sci. 2015; 56(2):778–786

[8] Gass JD, Blodi BA. Idiopathic juxtafoveolar retinal telangiectasis. Update of classification and follow-up study. Ophthalmology. 1993; 100(10):1536–1546

[9] Toto L, Di Antonio L, Mastropasqua R, et al. Multimodal imaging of macular telangiectasia type 2: focus on vascular changes using optical coherence tomography angiography. Invest Ophthalmol Vis Sci. 2016; 57(9):OCT268–OCT276

[10] Spaide RF, Klancnik JM, Jr, Cooney MJ. Retinal vascular layers in macular telangiectasia type 2 imaged by optical coherence tomographic angiography. JAMA Ophthalmol. 2015; 133(1): 66–73

[11] Zhang Q, Wang RK, Chen CL, et al. Swept Source optical coherence tomography angiography of neovascular macular telangiectasia type 2. Retina. 2015; 35(11):2285–2299

[12] Chidambara L, Gadde SG, Yadav NK, et al. Characteristics and quantification of vascular changes in macular telangiectasia type 2 on optical coherence tomography angiography. Br J Ophthalmol. 2016:bjophthalmol-2015–307941

[13] Roisman L, Rosenfeld PJ. Optical coherence tomography angiography of macular telangiectasia type 2. Dev Ophthalmol. 2016; 56:146–158

[14] Spaide RF, Klancnik JM, Jr, Cooney MJ, et al. Volume-rendering optical coherence tomography angiography of macular telangiectasia type 2. Ophthalmology. 2015; 122 (11):2261–2269

[15] Balaratnasingam C, Yannuzzi LA, Spaide RF. Possible choroidal neovascularization in macular telangiectasia type 2. Retina. 2015; 35(11):2317–2322

[16] Gaudric A, Krivosic V, Tadayoni R. Outer retina capillary invasion and ellipsoid zone loss in macular telangiectasia type 2 imaged by optical coherence tomography angiography. Retina. 2015; 35(11):2300–2306

[17] Thorell MR, Zhang Q, Huang Y, et al. Swept-source OCT angiography of macular telangiectasia type 2. Ophthalmic Surg Lasers Imaging Retina. 2014; 45(5):369–380

[18] Charbel Issa P, Heeren TF, Kupitz EH, Holz FG, Berendschot TT. Very early disease manifestations of macular telangiectasia type 2. Retina. 2016; 36(3):524–534

[19] Gillies MC, Mehta H, Bird AC. Macular telangiectasia type 2 without clinically detectable vasculopathy. JAMA Ophthalmol. 2015; 133(8):951–954

[20] Powner MB, Gillies MC, Zhu M, Vevis K, Hunyor AP, Fruttiger M. Loss of Müller's cells and photoreceptors in macular telangiectasia type 2. Ophthalmology. 2013; 120(11):2344–2352

[21] Scoles D, Flatter JA, Cooper RF, et al. Assessing photoreceptor structure associated with ellipsoid zone disruptions visualized with optical coherence tomography. Retina. 2016; 36(1):91–103

[22] Hasegawa E, Sweigard H, Husain D, et al. Characterization of a spontaneous retinal neovascular mouse model. PLoS One. 2014; 9(9):e106507

[23] Hu W, Jiang A, Liang J, et al. Expression of VLDLR in the retina and evolution of subretinal neovascularization in the knockout mouse model's retinal angiomatous proliferation. Invest Ophthalmol Vis Sci. 2008; 49(1):407–415

[24] Joyal JS, Sun Y, Gantner ML, et al. Retinal lipid and glucose metabolism dictates angiogenesis through the lipid sensor Ffar1. Nat Med. 2016; 22(4):439–445

[25] Zhao M, Andrieu-Soler C, Kowalczuk L, et al. A new CRB1 rat mutation links Müller glial cells to retinal telangiectasia. J Neurosci. 2015; 35(15):6093–6106

[26] Shen W, Fruttiger M, Zhu L, et al. Conditional Müller cell ablation causes independent neuronal and vascular pathologies in a novel transgenic model. J Neurosci. 2012; 32 (45):15715–15727

12 Optical Coherence Tomography Angiography and Adult-Onset Foveomacular Vitelliform Dystrophy

Giuseppe Querques, Adriano Carnevali, Federico Corvi, Lea Querques, Eric Souied, and Francesco Bandello

Summary

Optical coherence tomography angiography (OCTA) is a relatively new imaging technique that is becoming very useful in the diagnosis and follow-up of retinal diseases including adult-onset foveomacular vitelliform dystrophy (AFVD). Different OCTA plexa show nonspecific and specific alterations that correspond to the particular morphology of the vitelliform lesion. The simultaneous evaluation of other imaging techniques, such as infrared images, fundus autofluorescence (FAF), structural spectral-domain OCT (SD-OCT), fluorescein angiography, and indocyanine green angiography, is essential for the correct evaluation of OCTA images. Subfoveal choroidal neovascularization (CNV) may occur in few cases of AFVD. FAF, SD-OCT, and dye angiography remain the gold standard to assess the stage and for CNV diagnosis. Unfortunately, accumulation of yellowish subretinal material makes the diagnosis of CNV difficult, due to its masking effect and staining during dye angiography. Some recent studies have shown high sensitivity and specificity of OCTA in detecting CNV in AFVD patients. A correct interpretation of OCTA images may possibly be considered as a useful tool in guiding follow-up and treatment decision in AFVD disease.

Keywords: adult onset foveomacular vitelliform dystrophy, choroidal neovascularization, fluorescein angiography, fundus autofluorescence, indocyanine green angiography, macula, optical coherence tomography angiography, retinal imaging

12.1 Introduction

Adult-onset foveomacular vitelliform dystrophy (AFVD) is one of the most prevalent forms of macular degeneration.[1] AFVD has been included in the heterogeneous group of pattern dystrophy, in which the retinal pigment epithelium (RPE) is affected, along with butterfly-shaped pigment dystrophy, reticular dystrophy of the RPE, pseudo-Stargardt pattern dystrophy, and fundus pulverulentus.[2] It shares phenotypical features with best vitelliform macular dystrophy, but onset is in adult age, typically between the fourth and sixth decades.[1,3] It is a clinically heterogeneous and pleomorphic disease showing extreme variability in size, shape, and distribution of the subretinal deposition of yellowish material within the macula.[4,5,6] However, AFVD is not a monogenic disorder, and some of the genes involved, such as *PRPH2* or *BEST1*, are also involved in many other conditions such as Best disease, pattern dystrophies, or butterfly macular dystrophy.[7] Therefore, diagnosis of AFVD remains based on clinical features and imaging of the macula.[7]

12.2 Conventional Multimodal Imaging

A variety of imaging tools and functional analyses have been used to diagnose and study AFVD. Using structural spectral-domain optical coherence tomography (SD-OCT), the natural course of the disease has been classified into four stages: vitelliform (▶ Fig. 12.1, ▶ Fig. 12.2, ▶ Fig. 12.3, ▶ Fig. 12.4, ▶ Fig. 12.5, ▶ Fig. 12.6, ▶ Fig. 12.7, ▶ Fig. 12.8), pseudohypopyon (▶ Fig. 12.9), vitelliruptive (▶ Fig. 12.10), and atrophic stage, during which patients typically have slow progressive vision loss. In the vitelliform stage, structural SD-OCT shows dome-shaped subretinal homogeneously hyper-reflective material between RPE/Bruch's membrane and the ellipsoid zone (EZ) of the photoreceptors (▶ Fig. 12.1, ▶ Fig. 12.2, ▶ Fig. 12.3, ▶ Fig. 12.4, ▶ Fig. 12.5, ▶ Fig. 12.6, ▶ Fig. 12.7, ▶ Fig. 12.8). On infrared (IR) image, the vitelliform lesions appear as an inhomogeneous hyper-reflective zone (▶ Fig. 12.2 and ▶ Fig. 12.3); fundus autofluorescence (FAF) shows an increased signal that is not specific of AFVD (▶ Fig. 12.1, ▶ Fig. 12.2, ▶ Fig. 12.3, ▶ Fig. 12.4, ▶ Fig. 12.5, ▶ Fig. 12.6, ▶ Fig. 12.7, ▶ Fig. 12.8 and ▶ Fig. 12.10). The pseudohypopyon stage is characterized by the partial liquefaction of the lesion, corresponding, on structural SD-OCT, to a hyporeflective area in combination with a hyper-reflective homogeneous area containing the remaining vitelliform material (▶ Fig. 12.9). This hyporeflective material typically accumulates in the upper part of the lesion. Typically, the outer segment layers, overlying the liquefied area, present an irregular undersurface thickening representing deposits of nonphagocytized shed photoreceptor

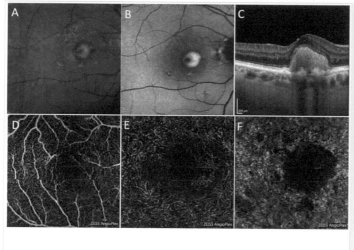

Fig. 12.1 Multicolor image, fundus autofluorescence (FAF), structural spectral-domain optical coherence tomography (SD-OCT), and OCT angiography (OCTA) of adult-onset foveomacular vitelliform dystrophy at the vitelliform stage. Multicolor image shows **(a)** central vitelliform material and FAF shows **(b)** central hyper-autofluorescence. **(c)** SD-OCT reveals the lesion as hyper-reflective material between retinal pigment epithelium/Bruch's membrane and the ellipsoid zone of the photoreceptors. On OCTA, the subretinal material leads to displacement of blood vessels at both the **(d)** superficial and **(e)** deep capillary plexus of the retina, associated with apparent vascular rarefaction at the **(f)** choriocapillaris.

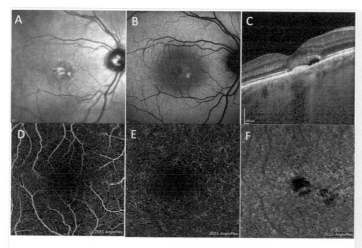

Fig. 12.2 Infrared (IR) reflectance, fundus autofluorescence (FAF), structural spectral-domain optical coherence tomography (SD-OCT), and OCT angiography (OCTA) of adult-onset foveomacular vitelliform dystrophy at the vitelliform stage. IR reflectance shows **(a)** mixed hyper-reflective/hyporeflective material and FAF shows **(b)** central hyper-autofluorescence/hypo-autofluorescence. SD-OCT **(c)** reveals the lesion as a hyper-reflective material between retinal pigment epithelium/Bruch's membrane and the ellipsoid zone of the photoreceptors with a small hyporeflective area that corresponds to an early resorption of vitelliform material. On OCTA, the subretinal material leads to displacement of blood vessels at both the **(d)** superficial and **(e)** deep capillary plexus of the retina, associated with apparent vascular rarefaction at the **(f)** choriocapillaris.

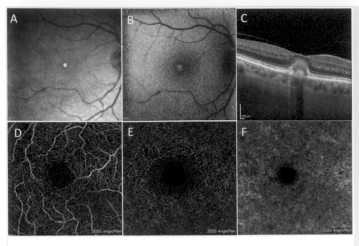

Fig. 12.3 Infrared (IR) reflectance, fundus autofluorescence (FAF), structural spectral-domain optical coherence tomography (SD-OCT), and OCT angiography (OCTA) of adult-onset foveomacular vitelliform dystrophy at the vitelliform stage. IR reflectance shows **(a)** mixed hyper-reflective/hyporeflective material and FAF shows **(b)** central hyper-autofluorescence/hypo-autofluorescence. SD-OCT **(c)** reveals the lesion as a hyper-reflective material between retinal pigment epithelium/Bruch's membrane and the ellipsoid zone of the photoreceptors with a small hyporeflective area that corresponds to an early resorption of vitelliform material. On OCTA, the subretinal material leads to displacement of blood vessels at both the **(d)** superficial and **(e)** deep capillary plexus of the retina, associated with apparent vascular rarefaction at the **(f)** choriocapillaris.

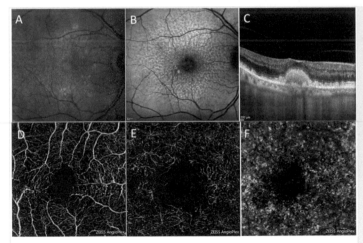

Fig. 12.4 Multicolor image, fundus autofluorescence (FAF), structural spectral-domain optical coherence tomography (SD-OCT), and OCT angiography (OCTA) of patient with pseudodrusen and adult-onset foveomacular vitelliform dystrophy at the vitelliform stage. Multicolor image shows **(a)** central vitelliform material and FAF **(b)** shows central hyper-autofluorescence with small circular hypofluorescent areas at the posterior pole. Structural SD-OCT reveals the lesion as hyper-reflective between retinal pigment epithelium/Bruch's membrane and the ellipsoid zone of the **(c)** photoreceptors with presence of pseudodrusen. On OCTA, the subretinal material leads to displacement of blood vessels at both the **(d)** superficial and **(e)** deep capillary plexus of the retina, associated with apparent vascular rarefaction at the **(f)** choriocapillaris.

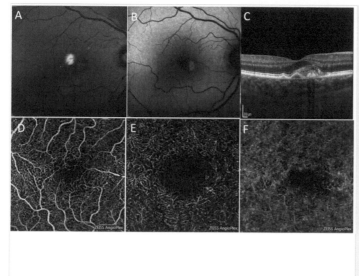

Fig. 12.5 Multicolor image, fundus autofluorescence (FAF), structural spectral-domain optical coherence tomography (SD-OCT), and OCT angiography (OCTA) of patient with pseudodrusen and adult-onset foveomacular vitelliform dystrophy at the vitelliform stage. Multicolor image shows **(a)** central vitelliform material and FAF **(b)** shows central hyper-autofluorescence with small circular hypofluorescent areas at the posterior pole. Structural SD-OCT reveals the lesion as hyper-reflective between retinal pigment epithelium/Bruch's membrane and the ellipsoid zone of the **(c)** photoreceptors with presence of pseudodrusen. On OCTA, the subretinal material leads to displacement of blood vessels at both the **(d)** superficial and **(e)** deep capillary plexus of the retina, associated with apparent vascular rarefaction at the **(f)** choriocapillaris.

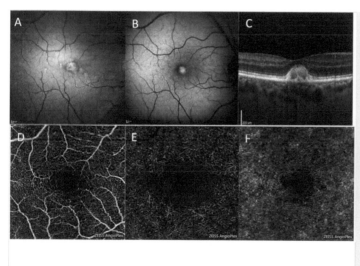

Fig. 12.6 Multicolor image, fundus autofluorescence (FAF), structural spectral-domain optical coherence tomography (SD-OCT), and OCT angiography (OCTA) of adult-onset foveomacular vitelliform dystrophy at the vitelliform stage. Multicolor image shows **(a)** central vitelliform material and FAF shows **(b)** central hyper-autofluorescence. SD-OCT reveals the lesion as hyper-reflective between retinal pigment epithelium/Bruch's membrane and the ellipsoid zone of the **(c)** photoreceptors. On OCTA, the subretinal material leads to displacement of blood vessels at both the **(d)** superficial and **(e)** deep capillary plexus of the retina, associated with apparent vascular rarefaction at the **(f)** choriocapillaris.

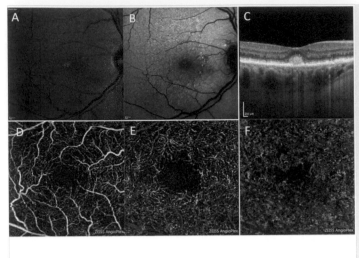

Fig. 12.7 Multicolor image, fundus autofluorescence (FAF), structural spectral-domain optical coherence tomography (SD-OCT), and OCT angiography (OCTA) of adult-onset foveomacular vitelliform dystrophy at the vitelliform stage. Multicolor image shows (a) central vitelliform material and (b) FAF shows central hyper-autofluorescence with small circular hypofluorescent areas at the posterior pole. Structural SD-OCT reveals the lesion as hyper-reflective between retinal pigment epithelium/Bruch's membrane and the ellipsoid zone of the (c) photoreceptors with presence of pseudodrusen. On OCTA, the subretinal material leads to displacement of blood vessels at both the (d) superficial and (e) deep capillary plexus of the retina, associated with apparent vascular rarefaction at the (f) choriocapillaris.

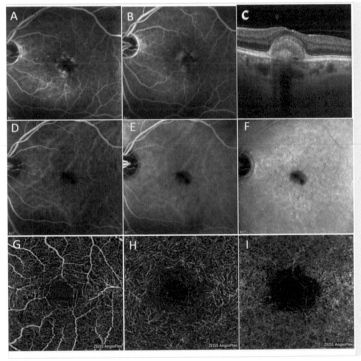

Fig. 12.8 Fluorescein angiography (FA), structural spectral-domain optical coherence tomography (SD-OCT), indocyanine green angiography (ICGA), and OCT angiography (OCTA) of adult-onset foveomacular vitelliform dystrophy at the vitelliform stage. Early FA phase reveals an inhomogeneous hyperfluorescence/hypofluorescence due to subretinal material accumulation, which turns into hyperfluorescent from the edges toward the center in (a,b) later phases. (c) SD-OCT shows central vitelliform material as a hyper-reflective lesion between retinal pigment epithelium/ Bruch's membrane and the ellipsoid zone of the photoreceptors. ICGA shows hypocyanescence in early, intermediate, and (d–f) late phases. On OCTA, the subretinal material leads to displacement of blood vessels at both the (g) superficial and the deep capillary plexus of the (h) retina, associated with apparent vascular rarefaction at the choriocapillaris (i).

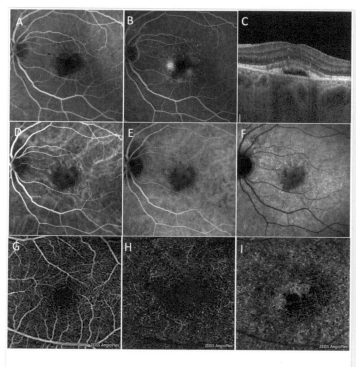

Fig. 12.9 Fluorescein angiography (FA), structural spectral-domain optical coherence tomography (SD-OCT), indocyanine green angiography (ICGA), and OCT angiography (OCTA) of adult-onset foveomacular vitelliform dystrophy at the pseudohypopyon stage. Early phase of FA reveals an inhomogeneous hyperfluorescence/hypofluorescence due to subretinal material accumulation, which turns into **(a,b)** hyperfluorescent from the edges toward the center in the late phase. **(c)** SD-OCT shows central vitelliform material as hyporeflective between retinal pigment epithelium/Bruch's membrane and the ellipsoid zone of the photoreceptors with some accumulation of hyper-reflective material on the borders. ICGA shows hypocyanescence in early, intermediate, and **(d–f)** late phases. On OCTA, the subretinal material leads to displacement of blood vessels at both the **(g)** superficial and **(h)** the deep capillary plexus of the retina, associated with apparent vascular rarefaction at the **(i)** choriocapillaris.

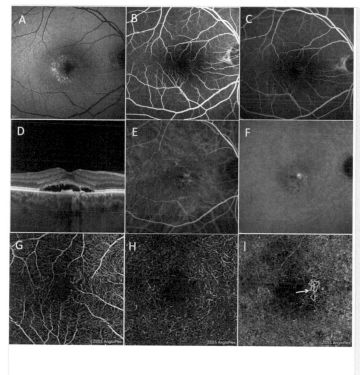

Fig. 12.10 Fundus autofluorescence (FAF), fluorescein angiography (FA), structural spectral-domain optical coherence tomography (SD-OCT), indocyanine green angiography (ICGA), and OCT angiography (OCTA) of adult-onset foveomacular vitelliform dystrophy at the vitelliruptive stage with choroidal neovascularization (CNV). FAF shows inhomogeneous accumulation of reflective/autofluorescent material in the **(a)** macular region. **(b,c)** FA and **(e,f)** ICGA show a hyperfluorescent area that increases in late phase (which is aspecific for CNV). **(d)** SD-OCT shows central vitelliform material as a hyporeflective lesion between retinal pigment epithelium/Bruch's membrane and the ellipsoid zone of the photoreceptors with some accumulation of hyper-reflective material in the outer surface of the retina. OCTA shows an incomplete foveal avascular zone in **(g)** the superficial and **(h)** deep capillary plexus, and a small CNV (*arrow*) with vascular rarefaction at the **(i)** choriocapillaris plexus.

outer segment material. In the vitelliruptive stage, the lesion flattens, much of the fluid is reabsorbed, and atrophy of the outer retina and RPE is evident (▸ Fig. 12.10). In the atrophic stage, the vitelliform material is completely reabsorbed resulting in the atrophy of the photoreceptor outer and inner segments, and atrophy of the outer nuclear layer and RPE. However, subfoveal choroidal neovascularization (CNV) may occur in few cases (▸ Fig. 12.10). Such complication occurs at an estimated rate of 11.7% after 6 years' follow-up.[8] Unfortunately, accumulation of yellowish subretinal material makes the diagnosis of CNV difficult, due to its masking effect.

On fluorescein angiography (FA), in the early stages of the disease, the vitelliform lesions may block the fluorescence due to the presence of vitelliform material and pigment in the fovea, often surrounded by a ring of defective transmission corresponding to an area of atrophied RPE. In the recirculation FA phase, staining of the vitelliform material by the fluorescein dye is often evident, and the staining pattern can be mistaken as occult type 1 CNV that may develop in eyes with AFVD.[9] In this case, a combination of clinical assessment and multimodal imaging such as indocyanine green angiography (ICGA) may be required in order to confirm or exclude the presence of CNV in addition to the vitelliform lesion (▸ Fig. 12.10).[9]

12.3 Optical Coherence Tomography Angiography

A relatively new imaging technique is optical coherence tomography angiography (OCTA) that allows noninvasive visualization of retinal and choroidal vasculature via motion contrast imaging. This tool maps erythrocyte movement over time by comparing sequential OCT B-scans at a given cross-section. Eye-tracking technology removes axial bulk motion from patient movement so that regions of motion between repeated OCT B-scans correspond to erythrocyte flow and, therefore, to vasculature. OCTA has the advantage not to require any dye injection and this permits achieving better and more detailed visualization of vascular networks without disturbance of dye leakage. There are several OCTA machines that use different algorithms to visualize blood flow and to allow detailed evaluation of the retinal microcirculation. In this series, we used the AngioPlex OCTA system (CIRRUS HD-OCT model 5000; Carl Zeiss Meditec, Inc., Dublin, CA) based on imaging contrast of optical microangiography (OMAG) image that evaluates the intrinsic optical scattering

signals backscattered by the moving blood cells in patent blood vessels. OMAG provides a unique ability to perform comprehensive measurements of the morphological and functional parameters of blood perfusion within a scanned tissue volume.[10,11] Angioplex CIRRUS HD-OCT model 5000 contains an A-scan rate of 68,000 scans per second, using a superluminescent diode centered on 840 nm. The resultant 3 × 3 angio cube contains 245 B-scan slices repeated up to × 4 at each B-scan position. Each B-scan is made of 245 A-scans and each A-scan is 1,024 pixels deep.

A 3 × 3 mm scanning area is the best pattern to ideally view the different retinal layers and to detect the presence of CNV. A manual adjustment on automatic segmentation provided by the machine software can be useful to ensure a correct visualization of the superficial and deep capillary plexus, avascular layer, and choriocapillaris layer.

Different OCTA plexa show alterations that correspond to the particular morphology of the vitelliform lesion, and the simultaneous evaluation of other imaging techniques (IR, FAF, SD-OCT, FA, ICGA) is essential for the correct assessment of OCTA images. The superficial and deep capillary plexus show, in most cases, a regular or irregular enlargement of the foveal avascular zone (FAZ) with small areas of reduced flow (black areas) especially around the FAZ (▸ Fig. 12.1, ▸ Fig. 12.2, ▸ Fig. 12.6, ▸ Fig. 12.8, and ▸ Fig. 12.9). In some cases, these vascular abnormalities are associated with the presence of long filamentous vessels running thorough the FAZ already described in the literature.[11] These vascular abnormalities may simply represent a coincident finding that presented in the vitelliform stage or these alterations could be the result of capillary reorganization due to long-lasting displacement of blood vessels at the superficial and deep capillary plexus of the retina. Of note, choriocapillaris plexus constantly shows a rarefaction of vascular network (▸ Fig. 12.1, ▸ Fig. 12.2, ▸ Fig. 12.3, ▸ Fig. 12.4, ▸ Fig. 12.5, ▸ Fig. 12.6, ▸ Fig. 12.7, ▸ Fig. 12.8, ▸ Fig. 12.9, ▸ Fig. 12.10). It is possible that the vascular rarefaction detected simply represented a suboptimal visualization of the different retinal and choroidal layers, due to masking from not only the hyperreflective, but also the hyporeflective subretinal material. Interestingly, in some cases, the OCTA can clearly show the presence of CNV (▸ Fig. 12.10), which is hardly visible on dye angiography, due to masking by vitelliform material (typically obscuring the visualization of neovascular network on both FA and ICGA).

12.4 Conclusion

This chapter describes the OCTA features of AFVD. OCTA is a new, noninvasive imaging that allows a fast and in vivo analysis of the morphology of both the superficial and deep capillary plexus, and choriocapillaris layer. In most cases of AFVD, the different OCTA vascular abnormalities visualized in the superficial and deep capillary plexus are occasional, nonspecific, and not related to the different stages of the disease. OCTA shows vascular network rarefaction with fewer blood vessels, nonperfused black areas around the FAZ, and regular or irregular enlargement of FAZ at the superficial and deep capillary plexus, and choriocapillaris layer. These vascular abnormalities may play a role in the pathogenesis or simply represent a consequence of material accumulation and reabsorption in AFVD. The most important utility of this new imaging technique in AFVD is the ability to properly visualize the presence of CNV that are hardly visible to normal FA or ICGA due to masking effect of the vitelliform material. Some recent studies have shown high sensitivity and specificity of OCTA in detecting CNV in AFVD patients.[11,12] Currently, FAF, SD-OCT, and dye angiography remain the gold standard to assess the stage and for CNV diagnosis, but OCTA may possibly be considered a useful tool in guiding follow-up and treatment decision in AFVD disease.

References

[1] Gass JD. A clinicopathologic study of a peculiar foveomacular dystrophy. Trans Am Ophthalmol Soc. 1974; 72:139–156

[2] Marmor MF, McNamara JA. Pattern dystrophy of the retinal pigment epithelium and geographic atrophy of the macula. Am J Ophthalmol. 1996; 122(3):382–392

[3] Gass JDM. Stereoscopic atlas of macular disease diagnosis and treatment. 4th ed. St Louis, MO: Mosby; 1997:303–325

[4] Vine AK, Schatz H. Adult-onset foveomacular pigment epithelial dystrophy. Am J Ophthalmol. 1980; 89(5):680–691

[5] Epstein GA, Rabb MF. Adult vitelliform macular degeneration: diagnosis and natural history. Br J Ophthalmol. 1980; 64(10): 733–740

[6] Gass JDM. Dominantly inherited adult form of vitelliform foveomacular dystrophy. In: Fine SL, Owens SL, eds. Management of retinal vascular and macular disorders. Baltimore, MD: Williams & Wilkins; 1983:182–186

[7] Chowers I, Tiosano L, Audo I, Grunin M, Boon CJ. Adult-onset foveomacular vitelliform dystrophy: A fresh perspective. Prog Retin Eye Res. 2015; 47:64–85

[8] Da Pozzo S, Parodi MB, Toto L, Ravalico G. Occult choroidal neovascularization in adult-onset foveomacular vitelliform dystrophy. Ophthalmologica. 2001; 215(6):412–414

[9] Querques G, Zambrowski O, Corvi F, et al. Optical coherence tomography angiography in adult-onset foveomacular vitelliform dystrophy. Br J Ophthalmol. 2016; 100(12):1724–1730

[10] Wang RK. Optical microangiography: a label free 3D imaging technology to visualize and quantify blood circulations within tissue beds in vivo. IEEE J Sel Top Quantum Electron. 2010; 16(3):545–554

[11] Wang RK, Jacques SL, Ma Z, Hurst S, Hanson SR, Gruber A. Three dimensional optical angiography. Opt Express. 2007; 15(7):4083–4097

[12] Lupidi M, Coscas G, Cagini C, Coscas F. Optical coherence tomography angiography of a choroidal neovascularization in adult onset foveomacular vitelliform dystrophy: pearls and pitfalls. Invest Ophthalmol Vis Sci. 2015; 56(13):7638–7645

13 Optical Coherence Tomography Angiography and High Myopia

Taku Wakabayashi and Yasushi Ikuno

Summary

In this chapter, we described the optical coherence tomography angiography (OCTA) findings in eyes with high myopia. The OCTA is especially useful in making diagnosis of myopic CNV noninvasively. The layer-specific imaging capabilities of OCTA may provide choriocapillaris changes in the area of progressive chorioretinal atrophy. Further advancement to obtain larger field of view and higher resolution of the deeper choroidal vasculature may have the potential to improve the diagnosis and evaluation of high myopia–related pathologies in the near future.

Keywords: high myopia, OCT angiography, optical coherence tomography angiography, choroidal neovascularization, chorioretinal atrophy

13.1 Introduction

High myopia, defined as spherical equivalent > 6 diopters (D) or axial length greater than 26.5 mm, is a major cause of visual impairment and blindness.[1,2,3,4] In high myopia, progressive elongation and deformation of the posterior segment may lead to the development of myopic macular lesions, including lacquer cracks, posterior staphyloma, choroidal neovascularization (CNV), macular hole retinal detachment, and chorioretinal atrophy. Vision-threatening pathology such as dome-shaped maculopathy and tilted-disc syndrome are also associated with high myopia.

Spectral-domain optical coherence tomography (SD-OCT) is widely used for noninvasive diagnosis and monitoring of abnormal chorioretinal morphology such as subretinal fluid associated with CNV, posterior staphyloma, and photoreceptor damage caused by chorioretinal atrophy.[5] Swept-source OCT (SS-OCT) has further improved the imaging beneath the retinal pigment epithelium (RPE) such as the choroid and the sclera by using a longer wavelength.[6,7] Fluorescein angiography (FA) is also an important diagnostic tool to evaluate myopic CNV in clinical practice. Leakage of the dye in the late phase is used to identify the presence and activity of the CNV. Indocyanine green angiography (ICGA) is another useful tool to evaluate the lacquer crack formation, choroidal blood flow, and extent of CNV lesion. Although those instruments are essential for the management of high myopia–related macular pathologies, the visualization of small retinal/choroidal vessels and the extent of CNV are sometimes difficult for the precise assessment.

OCT angiography (OCTA) is a new imaging modality that allows simultaneous visualization of vascular patterns of the choroidal and retinal vessels without the use of exogenous dyes.[8,9,10,11] The layer-specific imaging capabilities of OCTA have the potential to visualize both superficial and deep retinal capillary plexus, and the choriocapillaris by segmentation of each layer. Because it is difficult to visualize layer-specific vascular patterns by FA or ICGA, OCTA may provide a better understanding of pathogenesis and evaluation of treatment options for high myopia–related macular pathologies.

This chapter presents an overview of the OCTA findings in high myopia–related diseases and demonstrates the characteristics and clinical relevance of OCTA in high myopia.

13.2 Optical Coherence Tomography in High Myopia

▶ Fig. 13.1 shows OCTA images of the normal myopic macula taken by the RTVue XR Avanti (Optovue Inc, Fremont, CA) with AngioVue software. The 6 × 6 mm (▶ Fig. 13.1c–f) and 3 × 3 mm (▶ Fig. 13.1g–j) scanning areas centered on the fovea were obtained. The four en face images can be visualized on AngioVue mode, that is, superficial retina layer, deep retina layer, outer retina layer, and choriocapillaris layer. En face OCTA images show larger retinal vessels and capillaries in the superficial layer compared to the deep layer. As in healthy eyes without high myopia, the vascular density in the deep retinal layer in the highly myopic eyes is much higher than that in the superficial layer. In normal eyes, the outer retinal layer is devoid of blood vessels and flow signal is absent. Choriocapillaris layer shows dense microvascular structure within the choriocapillaris below the RPE.

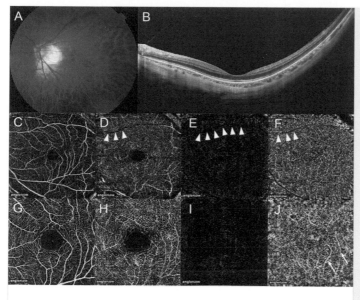

Fig. 13.1 optical coherence tomography angiography (OCTA) of a healthy 54-year-old male with high myopia. Normal myopic eye with axial length of 27.6 mm and spherical equivalent of −11 diopters. **(a)** Fundus photography. **(b)** B-scan spectral domain optical coherence tomography. **(c–f)** OCTA images of 6 × 6 mm centered on the fovea. **(c)** En face OCTA image of the superficial retinal layer, **(d)** deep retinal layer, **(e)** outer retina layer, and **(f)** choriocapillaris layer. **(d–f)** Arrowheads indicate shadowlike artifacts from superficial retinal vessels. **(g–j)** OCTA images of 3 × 3 mm centered on the fovea. **(g)** En face OCTA image of the superficial retinal layer, **(h)** deep retinal layer, **(i)** outer retina layer, and **(j)** choriocapillaris layer. **(j)** Arrows indicates superficial retinal vessels seen in choriocapillaris layer (projection artifacts).

13.3 Imaging Artifacts in High Myopia

The understanding of the imaging artifacts is important for accurate interpretation of the OCTA images.[12] First, the occasional eye motion causes motion artifacts on the OCTA image. Second, large superficial retinal vessels may result in lower signal below the vessels, which causes the shadowlike artifacts in the deep retinal layer, outer retinal layer, and the choriocapillaris layer (▶ Fig. 13.1d–f). The shadow artifacts are not part of the vasculature and may limit OCTA imaging on deeper structures. Third, projection artifacts, that is, superficial retinal vessels seen below, in deeper layers,[12] are often seen in highly myopic eyes compared with nonmyopic eyes (▶ Fig. 13.1j). The projection artifacts may limit the accurate quantitative assessment of vascular density in the deeper layer such as the choriocapillaris layer.

13.4 Myopic Choroidal Neovascularization

CNV is a major cause of severe visual loss in patients with pathologic myopia.[13] Myopic CNV occurs in 4 to 11% of patients with high myopia, with most of the eyes progressing to 20/200 or worse within 5 to 10 years after onset.[14,15] FA is the gold standard for diagnosing CNV; however, small CNV is sometimes obscured by transmitted hyperfluorescence due to surrounding chorioretinal atrophy and may limit identification of the active CNV lesion. In OCTA using RTVue XR Avanti with AngioVue software,[16] the CNV flow can be detected at the outer retinal layer between Bruch's membrane and the inner nuclear layer/outer plexiform layer junction (▶ Fig. 13.2). Because the outer retinal layer is devoid of blood vessels in normal subjects, flow signals at this layer strongly suggests CNV originating from the choroid (▶ Fig. 13.2c, h). The signal of the CNV network is more prominent in OCTA compared with FA or ICGA (▶ Fig. 13.2).

Intravitreal anti–vascular endothelial growth factor (anti-VEGF) therapy is the current standard therapy for myopic CNV.[17,18] Intravitreal anti-VEGF therapy has been used to improve both visual and anatomical outcomes. In OCTA, most of the CNV networks significantly attenuate after anti-VEGF therapy (▶ Fig. 13.3). However, small vascular networks usually remain even after exudation resolves on SD-OCT, indicating that blood flow does not completely disappear despite anti-VEGF therapy in myopic CNV. When the exudation reoccurs, OCTA may show evidence of re-enlarged vascular networks. Thus, OCTA is useful not only to monitor the efficacy of anti-VEGF treatment, but also to decide retreatment for recurrence.

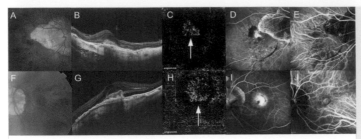

Fig. 13.2 Myopic choroidal neovascularization (CNV). **(a–e)** Case 1: an 87-year-old male patient with myopic CNV in the right eye. **(a)** Fundus photography shows subretinal hemorrhage. **(b)** Spectral-domain optical coherence tomography (SD-OCT) image shows subretinal fluid. **(c)** En face OCT angiography (3 × 3 mm) at the outer retinal layer shows CNV. The structure of the CNV network is much clearer compared to **(d)** fluorescein angiography or indocyanine angiography **(e)**. **(f–j)** Case 2: an 82-year-old male patient with myopic CNV in the left eye. **(f)** Fundus photograph shows yellowish lesion at the macula. **(g)** SD-OCT image shows subretinal fluid. **(h)** En face OCTA angiography (3 × 3 mm) at the outer retinal layer shows CNV. Large neovascular network is detected. Although the CNV lesion was detected by **(i)** fluorescein angiography and **(j)** indocyanine angiography, the precise structure was less identifiable.

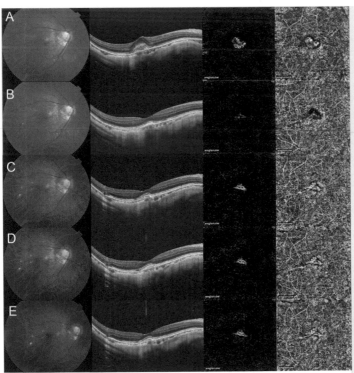

Fig. 13.3 optical coherence tomography angiography of myopic choroidal neovascularization (CNV) before and after anti–vascular endothelial growth factor (anti-VEGF) treatment. A 62-year-old female patient with myopic CNV in the right eye. Myopic CNV **(a)** before treatment and **(b)** 2 months, **(c)** 6 months, **(d)** 8 months, and **(e)** 10 months after anti-VEGF therapy. **(a)** Before treatment, fundus photography, optical coherence tomography (OCT) image, OCT angiography at the outer retinal layer, and OCT angiography at the choriocapillaris layer showing myopic CNV. Two consecutive anti-VEGF injections were performed. **(b)** Two months after anti-VEGF therapy, the OCT angiography at the outer retinal layer clearly showed a decreased size of the CNV. **(c)** Six months after initial treatment, OCT angiography showed slight enlargement of the CNV network, but without exudation on OCT. **(d)** Eight months after initial treatment, OCT angiography at the outer retinal layer showed stable CNV. **(e)** At 10 months, CNV structure remained stable without retreatment.

13.5 Lacquer Cracks

Lacquer cracks (LCs) present as a yellowish or white line in the posterior segment of pathologic myopia eyes. LCs are mechanical breaks in the choriocapillaris/RPE/Bruch's membrane due to progressive elongation of the posterior segment. LCs are more likely observed in eyes with myopic CNV; therefore, LCs have been considered a risk factor for myopic CNV.[19,20] In OCTA, the choriocapillaris flow at the area of the LCs shows normal pattern or, occasionally, partially disrupted pattern (▶ Fig. 13.4). In the case of partial disruption of the choriocapillaris layer on OCTA, the disruption may be due to a blocking effect by fibrous tissue or actual hypoperfusion of the choriocapillaris.

Further studies are required to elucidate the relation between LC formation and the choriocapillaris flow. Thus, in the current setting, OCTA may not provide crucial findings in the diagnosis or progression of LCs. However, OCTA can distinguish the presence or absence of CNV associated with newly developed subretinal hemorrhage at the LC lesion.

13.6 Chorioretinal Atrophy

Due to increased axial length and formation of posterior staphyloma, a variety of chorioretinal atrophy may develop in highly myopic eyes, such as diffuse atrophy, patchy atrophy, and macular atrophy.[21,22] ▶ Fig. 13.5 shows patchy chorioretinal atrophy

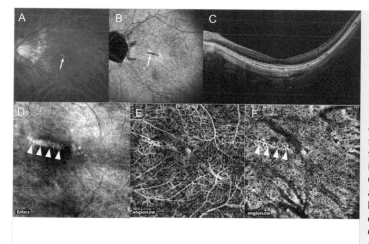

Fig. 13.4 Lacquer cracks. A 48-year old female patient with lacquer cracks (LCs). The patient had axial length of 29.8 mm and previous history of simple retinal hemorrhage. **(a)** Fundus photography shows yellowish line indicating LCs formation. **(b)** The late phase indocyanine green angiography confirms LC formation. **(c)** Swept-source OCT B-scan image. **(d)** Full-thickness en face image showing the LCs (arrowheads). **(e)** Full-thickness OCT angiography (3 × 3 mm). **(f)** OCT angiography at the choriocapillaris layer shows possible partial disruption of the choriocapillaris without choroidal neovascularization associated with LCs (arrowheads).

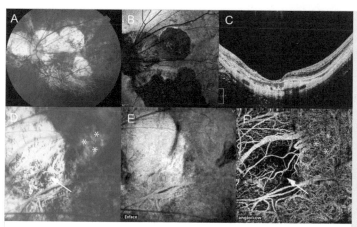

Fig. 13.5 Chorioretinal atrophy. A 54- year old female patient with axial length of 33.2 mm. **(a)** Fundus photography shows patchy chorioretinal atrophy within diffuse chorioretinal atrophy. **(b)** Autofluorescence image shows hypofluorescence associated with patchy atrophy. **(c)** Swept-source optical coherence tomography (SD-OCT) image. **(d)** Magnification of the fundus photograph showing the area of patchy atrophy (arrow) and diffuse atrophy (asterisk). **(e)** Corresponding en face OCT image. **(f)** En face OCT angiography image at the choriocapillaris layer shows defect of choriocapillaris flow in the area of patchy atrophy and preserved choriocapillaris flow in the area of diffuse atrophy (asterisk).

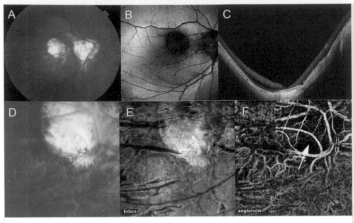

Fig. 13.6 Macular atrophy. A 55-year old male with axial length of 30.7 mm. The visual acuity was 20/20.
(a) Fundus photography shows chorioretinal atrophy at the macula (macular atrophy).
(b) Autofluorescence image shows hypofluorescence associated with macular atrophy. (c) Swept-source optical coherence tomography (OCT) image shows significant posterior staphyloma and thinning of choroid and retina at the macula.
(d) Magnification of the fundus photograph. (e) Corresponding en face OCT image. (f) En face OCT angiography image at the choriocapillaris layer shows defect of the choriocapillaris flow in the area of macular atrophy (arrow). Large choroidal vessels are still visible.

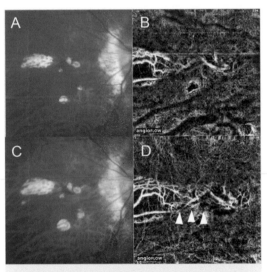

Fig. 13.7 Progression of chorioretinal atrophy.
(a) Fundus photography shows patchy chorioretinal atrophy around the fovea. (b) Optical coherence tomography (OCT) angiography image (choriocapillaris layer). (c) One and half years later, chorioretinal atrophy seems to extend toward the fovea. (d) OCT angiography image (choriocapillaris layer) shows progressive disruption of choriocapillaris (arrowheads).

within the area of diffuse chorioretinal atrophy. Fundus photograph shows grayish-white, well-demarcated atrophy in the area of patchy atrophy. On OCTA, choriocapillaris flow is lost, but relatively large choroidal vessels remain in the area of patchy

atrophy (► Fig. 13.5f). On the other hand, choriocapillaris flow seems to be preserved on OCTA in the area of diffuse chorioretinal atrophy.

► Fig. 13.6 shows macular atrophy. On OCTA, the area of macular atrophy is associated with loss of choriocapillaris flow, indicating the lack of choriocapillaris layer. The progression of the chorioretinal atrophy is associated with enlargement of the choriocapillaris loss on OCTA as shown in ► Fig. 13.7.

Reference

[1] Iwase A, Araie M, Tomidokoro A, Yamamoto T, Shimizu H, Kitazawa Y, Tajimi Study Group. Prevalence and causes of low vision and blindness in a Japanese adult population: the Tajimi Study. Ophthalmology. 2006; 113(8):1354–1362

[2] Klaver CC, Wolfs RC, Vingerling JR, Hofman A, de Jong PT. Age-specific prevalence and causes of blindness and visual impairment in an older population: the Rotterdam Study. Arch Ophthalmol. 1998; 116(5):653–658

[3] Hsu WM, Cheng CY, Liu JH, Tsai SY, Chou P. Prevalence and causes of visual impairment in an elderly Chinese population in Taiwan: the Shihpai Eye Study. Ophthalmology. 2004; 111 (1):62–69

[4] Xu L, Wang Y, Li Y, et al. Causes of blindness and visual impairment in urban and rural areas in Beijing: the Beijing Eye Study. Ophthalmology. 2006; 113(7):1134.e1–1134.e11

[5] Ikuno Y, Jo Y, Hamasaki T, Tano Y. Ocular risk factors for choroidal neovascularization in pathologic myopia. Invest Ophthalmol Vis Sci. 2010; 51(7):3721–3725

[6] Ohno-Matsui K, Akiba M, Ishibashi T, Moriyama M. Observations of vascular structures within and posterior to sclera in eyes with pathologic myopia by swept-source optical coherence tomography. Invest Ophthalmol Vis Sci. 2012; 53(11):7290–7298

[7] Asai T, Ikuno Y, Akiba M, Kikawa T, Usui S, Nishida K. Analysis of peripapillary geometric characters in high myopia using swept-source optical coherence tomography. Invest Ophthalmol Vis Sci. 2016; 57(1):137–144

[8] Kim DY, Fingler J, Zawadzki RJ, et al. Optical imaging of the chorioretinal vasculature in the living human eye. Proc Natl Acad Sci USA. 2013; 110(35):14354–14359

[9] Choi W, Mohler KJ, Potsaid B, et al. Choriocapillaris and choroidal microvasculature imaging with ultrahigh speed OCT angiography. PLoS One. 2013; 8(12):e81499

[10] Schwartz DM, Fingler J, Kim DY, et al. Phase-variance optical coherence tomography: a technique for noninvasive angiography. Ophthalmology. 2014; 121(1):180–187

[11] Spaide RF, Klancnik JM, Jr, Cooney MJ. Retinal vascular layers imaged by fluorescein angiography and optical coherence tomography angiography. JAMA Ophthalmol. 2015; 133(1): 45–50

[12] Spaide RF, Fujimoto JG, Waheed NK. Image artifacts in optical coherence tomography angiography. Retina. 2015; 35(11): 2163–2180

[13] Soubrane G, Coscas GJ. Choroidal neovascular membrane in degenerative myopia. In: Ryan SJ, ed. Retina. 4th ed. St. Louis, MO: Mosby; 2005:1136–1152

[14] Avila MP, Weiter JJ, Jalkh AE, Trempe CL, Pruett RC, Schepens CL. Natural history of choroidal neovascularization in degenerative myopia. Ophthalmology. 1984; 91(12):1573–1581

[15] Yoshida T, Ohno-Matsui K, Yasuzumi K, et al. Myopic choroidal neovascularization: a 10-year follow-up. Ophthalmology. 2003; 110(7):1297–1305

[16] Miyata M, Ooto S, Hata M, et al. Detection of myopic choroidal neovascularization using optical coherence tomography angiography. Am J Ophthalmol. 2016; 165:108–114

[17] Sakaguchi H, Ikuno Y, Gomi F, et al. Intravitreal injection of bevacizumab for choroidal neovascularisation associated with pathological myopia. Br J Ophthalmol. 2007; 91(2):161–165

[18] Ikuno Y, Ohno-Matsui K, Wong TY, et al. MYRROR Investigators. Intravitreal aflibercept injection in patients with myopic choroidal neovascularization: the MYRROR study. Ophthalmology. 2015; 122(6):1220–1227

[19] Ikuno Y, Sayanagi K, Soga K, et al. Lacquer crack formation and choroidal neovascularization in pathologic myopia. Retina. 2008; 28(8):1124–1131

[20] Ohno-Matsui K, Yoshida T, Futagami S, et al. Patchy atrophy and lacquer cracks predispose to the development of choroidal neovascularization in pathological myopia. Br J Ophthalmol. 2003; 87(5):570–573

[21] Curtin BJ, Karlin DB. Axial length measurements and fundus changes of the myopic eye. I. The posterior fundus. Trans Am Ophthalmol Soc. 1970; 68:312–334

[22] Ohno-Matsui K, Kawasaki R, Jonas JB, et al. META-analysis for Pathologic Myopia (META-PM) Study Group. International photographic classification and grading system for myopic maculopathy. Am J Ophthalmol. 2015; 159(5):877–83.e7

14 Optical Coherence Tomography Angiography and Uveitis

Eduardo A. Novais, André Romano, and Rubens Belfort Jr.

Summary

Many imaging modalities have been used for the diagnosis and follow-up of patients with uveitis, and to identify and monitor the development of visually debilitating sequelae, such as vasculitis, retinal and choroidal neovascularization, and cystoid macular edema. Fluorescein and indocyanine green angiography are the gold standard techniques to evaluate retinal vascular occlusion disease and choroidal neovascularization, two severe complications in uveitis. However, these imaging modalities are invasive, involving the use of an intravenous dye that can result in systemic side effects and anaphylaxis. Optical coherence tomography angiography (OCTA) is a noninvasive, depth-resolved imaging modality that allows for the appreciation of spatial relationships of fundus vessels and enables detailed en face visualization of the retinal and choroidal vasculature separately without the risk of adverse effects associated with the administration of intravenous dye. OCTA has some distinct advantages compared to dye-based angiography for analysis of retinal and choroidal vascular diseases such as retinal vascular occlusions and choroidal neovascularization secondary to posterior uveitis, including its rapid and comfortable image acquisition, depth resolution, lack of a need of invasive dye injection, assessment of the retinal capillary networks at different depths and better quantification of retinal ischemia.

Keywords: posterior uveitis, retinal vasculitis, choroidal neovascularization, optical coherence tomography

14.1 Introduction

Uveitis is an umbrella term for a variety of inflammatory eye conditions. It is a major cause of severe visual impairment worldwide and affects not only the uvea but also the retina, optic nerve, and the vitreous.[1] The etiology may be idiopathic or secondary to various infectious, neoplastic, or autoimmune diseases. Currently, many imaging modalities, such as color fundus photography, fluorescein angiography (FA), indocyanine green angiography (ICGA), optical coherence tomography (OCT), and fundus autofluorescence (FAF) have been used for the diagnosis and follow-up of patients with uveitis.[2,3,4,5,6,7,8] These imaging modalities can be used to identify and monitor the development of visually debilitating sequelae, such as vasculitis, retinal and choroidal neovascularization, and cystoid macular edema (CME).[3,4,5,9] The gold standard techniques, FA and ICGA, are not perfect given they are invasive, involving the use of intravenous dye that can result in systemic side effects and rarely anaphylaxis.[10,11,12]

Unlike FA and ICGA, OCT angiography (OCTA) is a noninvasive, depth-resolved imaging modality that allows for the appreciation of spatial relationships of fundus vessels and enables detailed en face visualization of the retinal and choroidal vasculature separately without the risk of adverse effects associated with the administration of intravenous dye.[13,14] OCTA uses signal decorrelation between consecutive transverse cross-sectional OCT scans.[15] An OCTA image is computed by comparing, on a pixel-by-pixel basis, repeated B-scans acquired at the same retinal location in rapid succession. The rationale behind OCTA imaging is that in static nonmobile tissue, the reflected signal will be stationary, thus the repeated B-scans will be identical. Inside vasculature, moving erythrocytes cause a time-dependent backscattering of the OCT signal, so that the repeated B-scans are not identical.[13,14,16] This change between the sequential B-scans can be processed to provide an OCTA scan. Areas of flow are noted as white and areas of no flow are seen as black. Previous studies have shown that the 3×3 mm OCT angiograms can visualize greater vascular detail compared to FA or ICGA.[17,18] Importantly, OCT angiograms can also be viewed alongside corresponding structural en face and OCT B-scans, which can be used to visualize increased central retinal thickness and intraretinal cysts and correlate these structural findings to microvascular details.

14.2 Optical Coherence Tomography Angiography in Retinal Vasculitis

Retinal vasculitis is a sight-threatening complication that can be present in many systemic autoimmune, inflammatory, and infectious diseases such as sarcoidosis, Behçet's disease, lupus, multiple sclerosis, birdshot chorioretinopathy, cytomegalovirus, and many others.[19,20,21,22,23] On clinical examination, retinal vasculitis presents as vascular sheathing, cotton wool spots, retinal hemorrhages, and vein occlusions that can lead to secondary retinal ischemia, neovascularization of the retina and optic disc, and CME.[24] These features are often well demonstrated by FA, which has been the gold standard to evaluate disease activity and subsequent adverse events. This imaging modality can easily identify leakage from the vasculature wall secondary to a breakdown of the blood–retinal barrier, areas of ischemia, and retinal and optic disc neovascularization.[25]

The retinal capillary network is arranged in distinct layers and are connected by perpendicularly positioned vessels.[26] The capillaries from the superficial retinal plexus are located predominantly within the ganglion cell layer, whereas the capillaries from the deep retinal plexus are located at the outer boundary of the inner nuclear layer, with a smaller intermediate retinal capillary plexus at the inner margin of the inner nuclear layer. Previous studies showed that these two retinal capillary plexuses could be disproportionately affected by a retinal vascular disease, and the deep vascular plexus often presents a more prominent decreased flow.[18,27] However, since dye-based angiography is only able to visualize the retinal vasculature using two-dimensional imaging, independent evaluation of those plexuses was only possible with the advent of the depth-resolved capability of OCTA. Patients with retinal occlusion who are often noted to have areas of ischemic capillary nonperfusion on FA have recently been correlated with areas of retinal nonperfusion on OCT angiograms.[28] In occlusive vasculitis, OCTA imaging highlights that the vessels can become tortuous, narrowed, and focally dilated. Truncated vessels can also be present on OCT angiograms with abrupt interruptions and focal terminal dilations at the site of the occlusion. Vascular looping and telangiectatic vessels that are often obscured by dye leakage on FA can also be easily visualized with OCTA.[29]

Another important feature of OCTA is the ability to automatically evaluate some quantitative vascular features such as vessel density and flow indices (▶ Fig. 14.1).[30,31] Additionally, the combination of blood flow analysis obtained by OCT angiograms

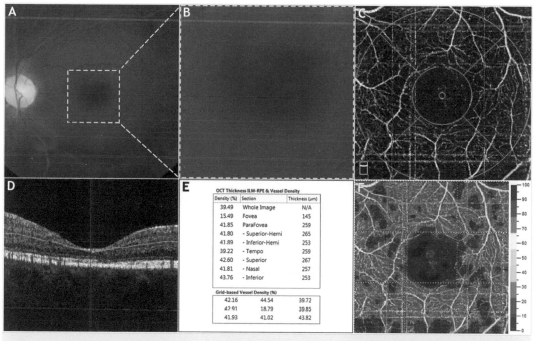

Fig. 14.1 Quantitative analysis of the vascular density using optical coherence tomography angiography (OCTA) of the left eye of a 46-year-old female patient with retinal vasculitis secondary to Behçet's disease. (a) Color fundus photography shows diffuse retinal atrophy associated with vascular sheathing and tortuosity. (b) Yellow dashed frame identifies the corresponding 3 × 3 mm area imaged on OCTA. (c) En face OCTA segmented at the level of the superficial retinal plexus. (d) Corresponding OCT B-scan segmentation of the superficial plexus with decorrelation signal overlay. (e) Quantitative analysis of the retinal thickness (μm) and vascular density (%). (f) Superficial capillary plexus map shows a mild decrease of the vascular density (39.49%).

to the structural en face and OCT B-scans makes this imaging modality a useful tool for evaluating progression of disease and response to treatment in retinal vasculitis.

The disadvantage of OCTA in retinal vasculitis is the inability to detect vascular sheathing, an important sign that can be easily seen on dye-based angiography. This vascular leakage is not visualized by OCTA for two reasons. First, because retinal vasculitis is associated with leukocytes extravasation into the extravascular space,[32] not erythrocytes, and this leaking fluid does not strongly backscatter the incident OCT beam. Second, the relatively low leakage flux in retinal vasculitis means that even if the fluid did appreciably backscatter the OCT beam, the flux would not be detectable with OCTA, which is typically sensitive to backscatters with speeds in the millimeter per second range (► Fig. 14.2).

14.3 Optical Coherence Tomography Angiography in Chorioretinal Inflammations

The greatest advantage of OCTA compared to previous imaging modalities in posterior uveitis is the ability to noninvasively monitor these patients for potential complications such as choroidal neovascularization (CNV), which can be associated with severe visual loss.

14.3.1 White Dot Syndromes

White dot syndromes (WDS) are a group of inflammatory chorioretinal diseases characterized by the presence of yellowish-white lesions. Those lesions can affect the choroid, retinal pigment epithelium (RPE), and retina.[33] The WDS spectrum includes birdshot chorioretinopathy, serpiginous

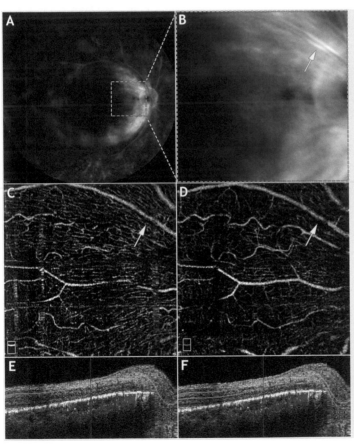

Fig. 14.2 Multimodal imaging of the left eye of a 46-year-old female patient with retinal vasculitis secondary to Behçet's disease. (a) Fluorescein angiography (FA) shows a diffuse background hyperfluorescence associated with vascular sheathing. (b) Yellow dashed frame identifies the corresponding 3 × 3 mm area imaged on optical coherence tomography angiography (OCTA). The yellow arrow points the area of vascular sheathing. (c,d) En face OCTA segmented at the level of the superficial and deep retinal plexuses, respectively. OCTA did not reproduce the same FA finding. (e,f) represents corresponding OCT B-scans segmentation of the superficial and deep plexuses, respectively, with decorrelation signal overlay.

choroiditis, multifocal choroiditis (MFC), punctate inner choroidopathy (PIC), and acute zonal occult outer retinopathy (AZOOR). Symptoms may include mild to severe decrease in visual acuity that can often be associated with visual field defects and photopsia. The use of multimodal imaging has guided the diagnosis and treatment through the use of FAF, FA, ICGA, and structural OCT B-scans.[5,6,34]

Previous reports have shown that OCTA could detect choriocapillaris flow impairment in birdshot chorioretinopathy besides the aforementioned retinal vascular disorders.[35] In acute serpiginous choroiditis, markedly increased thickness and decreased circulation in the choroid has been described.[36] OCTA can detect reduced choriocapillaris flow in these patients. However, this finding needs to be cautiously evaluated since the sub-RPE plaques present in this phase can block the OCT signal, leading to a misdiagnosis of flow impairment. In patients with Zone 3 (choroidal atrophy) AZOOR, OCTA depicts a choriocapillaris impairment. In MFC and PIC, OCTA becomes crucial as it allows for the early detection of secondary CNV.

14.3.2 OCT Angiography for Secondary Choroidal Neovascularization

Perhaps one of the most important applications of this imaging modality is the possibility to early detect CNV as an adverse event of posterior uveitis (toxoplasmosis, serpiginous choroiditis, MFC, PIC, etc.; ▶ Fig. 14.3 and ▶ Fig. 14.4).[37] This sight-threating complication demands a correct and early diagnosis for prompt intraocular anti–vascular endothelial growth factor treatment.[38] Evaluation of CNV using OCTA has been extensively described and is one of the most important applications of this modality.[16,39,40] Depending on the clinical presentation, OCTA sensitivity to visualize abnormal vascular network may vary. The CNV complex can often be identified as abnormal choroidal vessels that correspond to a distinct, high-flow, tangled irregular filamentous vascular network in the outer retinal, choriocapillaris, or in both layers.[41] When a massive hemorrhage, exudate, or fibrotic tissue is present, OCTA signals can be blocked, decreasing visualization. Because CNV

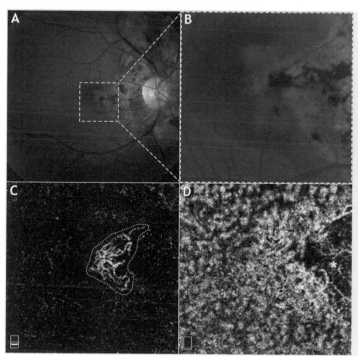

Fig. 14.3 Multimodal imaging of the right eye of a 30-year-old female patient with choroidal neovascularization (CNV) secondary to serpiginous choroiditis. **(a)** Color fundus photography shows a peripapillary chorioretinal atrophy. **(b)** Yellow dashed frame identifies the corresponding 3 × 3 mm area imaged on optical coherence tomography angiography (OCTA). **(c)** En face OCTA segmented at the level of the outer retina shows a distinct and filamentous CNV (yellow dotted line). **(d)** En face OCTA segmented at the level of the choriocapillaris shows an area of absence of flow that corresponds to the chorioretinal atrophy area (yellow asterisk).

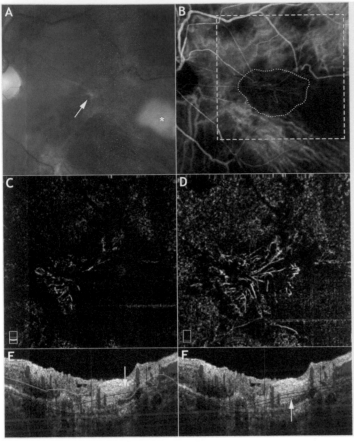

Fig. 14.4 Multimodal imaging of the left eye of a 65-year-old male patient with choroidal neovascularization (CNV) secondary to toxoplasmosis retinochoroiditis. **(a)** Color fundus photography shows a fibrotic tissue contraction (white arrow) associated with a hypochromic nonexudative lesion (white asterisk). **(b)** Indocyanine green angiography identifies a CNV (white dotted line). Yellow dashed line represents the 6 × 6 mm area imaged on optical coherence tomography angiography (OCTA). **(c,d)** represent en face OCTA of the outer retina and choriocapillaris, respectively, showing a distinct and filamentous CNV. **(e,f)** represent corresponding OCT B-scans segmentation of the outer retina and choriocapillaris, respectively, identifying a segmentation error secondary to abnormal retinal architecture (yellow arrows).

secondary to posterior uveitis is rarely associated with massive subretinal hemorrhages that limit penetration of OCT signal, the abnormal vascular network may be identified with a screening OCTA in such cases.

14.4 Disadvantages of Optical Coherence Tomography Angiography in Uveitis

In cases where significant retinal atrophy or macular edema causes distortion of the retinal architecture, the automated segmentation of the retinal layers becomes challenging and less accurate (▶ Fig. 14.4e, f). An apparent decrease in vascular perfusion is more prominent in patients with macular edema; however, this may be caused due to signal attenuation secondary to the shadowing effect of the fluid accumulation, or due to displacement of vessels by fluid, thus leading to a potential overestimation of the degree of decreased vascular perfusion. In addition, OCTA has limited field of view, inability to view leakage, increased potential for artifacts (blink, movement), and inability to detect blood flow below the slowest threshold flow.

14.5 Conclusion

Further improvement of OCTA is still required for this imaging modality to have a role in a daily clinical application that is comparable to that of FA. However, there are some distinct advantages of OCTA compared to dye-based angiography for analysis of retinal and choroidal vascular diseases such as retinal vasculitis and CNV secondary to posterior uveitis, including its rapid and comfortable image acquisition, depth resolution, lack of a need of invasive dye injection, assessment of the retinal capillary networks at different depths, and better quantification of retinal ischemia. An absence of dynamic blood flow at the capillary level and vascular leakage information, which conventional FA can provide, are significant limitations. In time, with the development of OCTA, OCT as a single modality can provide most of the multidimensional information needed to manage patients with uveitis. As this new technology improves, it is hoped that it may remove the need for invasive techniques such as dye injection in the investigation and management of patients with uveitis.

References

[1] Miserocchi E, Fogliato G, Modorati G, Bandello F. Review on the worldwide epidemiology of uveitis. Eur J Ophthalmol. 2013; 23(5):705–717

[2] Kim JS, Knickelbein JE, Jaworski L, et al. Enhanced depth imaging optical coherence tomography in uveitis: an intravisit and interobserver reproducibility study. Am J Ophthalmol. 2016; 164:49–56

[3] Onal S, Tugal-Tutkun I, Neri P, P Herbort C. Optical coherence tomography imaging in uveitis. Int Ophthalmol. 2014; 34(2):401–435

[4] Bhaleeya SD, Davis J. Imaging retinal vascular changes in uveitis. Int Ophthalmol Clin. 2012; 52(4):83–96

[5] Herbort CP, Mantovani A, Papadia M. Use of indocyanine green angiography in uveitis. Int Ophthalmol Clin. 2012; 52(4):13–31

[6] Spaide RF, Goldberg N, Freund KB. Redefining multifocal choroiditis and panuveitis and punctate inner choroidopathy through multimodal imaging. Retina. 2013; 33(7):1315–1324

[7] Finamor LP, Muccioli C, Belfort R, Jr. Imaging techniques in the diagnosis and management of uveitis. Int Ophthalmol Clin. 2005; 45(2):31–40

[8] Lavinsky D, Romano A, Muccioli C, Belfort R, Jr. Imaging in ocular toxoplasmosis. Int Ophthalmol Clin. 2012; 52(4):131–143

[9] Palácio GL, Gabbai AA, Muccioli C, Belfort R, Jr. Images in medicine. Occlusion of the central vein of the retina after treatment with intravenous human immunoglobulin. Rev Assoc Med Bras (1992). 2004; 50(3):246

[10] Ha SO, Kim DY, Sohn CH, Lim KS. Anaphylaxis caused by intravenous fluorescein: clinical characteristics and review of literature. Intern Emerg Med. 2014; 9(3):325–330

[11] Musa F, Muen WJ, Hancock R, Clark D. Adverse effects of fluorescein angiography in hypertensive and elderly patients. Acta Ophthalmol Scand. 2006; 84(6):740–742

[12] Garski TR, Staller BJ, Hepner G, Banka VS, Finney RA, Jr. Adverse reactions after administration of indocyanine green. JAMA. 1978; 240(7):635

[13] Jonathan E, Enfield J, Leahy MJ. Correlation mapping method for generating microcirculation morphology from optical coherence tomography (OCT) intensity images. J Biophotonics. 2011; 4(9):583–587

[14] An L, Wang RK. In vivo volumetric imaging of vascular perfusion within human retina and choroids with optical micro-angiography. Opt Express. 2008; 16(15):11438–11452

[15] Lumbroso BHD, Jia Y, Fujimoto JA, Rispoli M. Diabetic retinopathy. In Clinical Guide to Angio-OCT. New Delhi: Jaypee Brothers; 2014:35–44

[16] de Carlo TE, Bonini Filho MA, Chin AT, et al. Spectral-domain optical coherence tomography angiography of choroidal neovascularization. Ophthalmology. 2015; 122(6):1228–1238

[17] Matsunaga D, Yi J, Puliafito CA, Kashani AH. OCT angiography in healthy human subjects. Ophthalmic Surg Lasers Imaging Retina. 2014; 45(6):510–515

[18] Kashani AH, Lee SY, Moshfeghi A, Durbin MK, Puliafito CA. Optical coherence tomography angiography of retinal venous occlusion. Retina. 2015; 35(11):2323–2331

[19] Talat L, Lightman S, Tomkins-Netzer O. Ischemic retinal vasculitis and its management. J Ophthalmol. 2014; 2014:197675

[20] Yen YC, Weng SF, Chen HA, Lin YS. Risk of retinal vein occlusion in patients with systemic lupus erythematosus: a population-based cohort study. Br J Ophthalmol. 2013; 97(9):1192–1196

[21] Tugal-Tutkun I, Onal S, Altan-Yaycioglu R, Huseyin Altunbas H, Urgancioglu M. Uveitis in Behçet disease: an analysis of 880 patients. Am J Ophthalmol. 2004; 138(3):373–380

[22] Lightman S, McDonald WI, Bird AC, et al. Retinal venous sheathing in optic neuritis. Its significance for the pathogenesis of multiple sclerosis. Brain. 1987; 110(Pt 2):405–414

[23] Herbort CP, Rao NA, Mochizuki M, members of Scientific Committee of First International Workshop on Ocular Sarcoidosis. International criteria for the diagnosis of ocular sarcoidosis: results of the first International Workshop On Ocular Sarcoidosis (IWOS). Ocul Immunol Inflamm. 2009; 17(3):160–169

[24] Levy-Clarke GA, Nussenblatt R. Retinal vasculitis. Int Ophthalmol Clin. 2005; 45(2):99–113

[25] Rosenbaum JT, Sibley CH, Lin P. Retinal vasculitis. Curr Opin Rheumatol. 2016; 28(3):228–235

[26] Snodderly DM, Weinhaus RS, Choi JC. Neural-vascular relationships in central retina of macaque monkeys (Macaca fascicularis). J Neurosci. 1992; 12(4):1169–1193

[27] Sarraf D, Rahimy E, Fawzi AA, et al. Paracentral acute middle maculopathy: a new variant of acute macular neuroretinopathy associated with retinal capillary ischemia. JAMA Ophthalmol. 2013; 131(10):1275–1287

[28] Kuehlewein L, An L, Durbin MK, Sadda SR. Imaging areas of retinal nonperfusion in ischemic branch retinal vein occlusion with swept-source OCT microangiography. Ophthalmic Surg Lasers Imaging Retina. 2015; 46(2):249–252

[29] Novais EA, Adhi M, Moult EM, et al. Choroidal neovascularization analyzed on ultrahigh-speed swept-source optical coherence tomography angiography compared to spectral-domain optical coherence tomography angiography. Am J Ophthalmol. 2016; 164:80–88

[30] Huang D, Jia Y, Gao SS, Lumbroso B, Rispoli M. Optical coherence tomography angiography using the optovue device. Dev Ophthalmol. 2016; 56:6–12

[31] Hwang TS, Gao SS, Liu L, et al. Automated quantification of capillary nonperfusion using optical coherence tomography angiography in diabetic retinopathy. JAMA Ophthalmol. 2016; 134(4):367–373

[32] Crane IJ, Liversidge J. Mechanisms of leukocyte migration across the blood-retina barrier. Semin Immunopathol. 2008; 30(2):165–177

[33] Crawford CM, Igboeli O. A review of the inflammatory chorioretinopathies: the white dot syndromes. ISRN Inflamm. 2013; 2013:783190

[34] Bansal R, Gupta A, Gupta V. Imaging in the diagnosis and management of serpiginous choroiditis. Int Ophthalmol Clin. 2012; 52(4):229–236

[35] de Carlo TE, Bonini Filho MA, Adhi M, Duker JS. Retinal and choroidal vasculature in birdshot chorioretinopathy analyzed using spectral domain optical coherence tomography angiography. Retina. 2015; 35(11):2392–2399

[36] Takahashi A, Saito W, Hashimoto Y, Saito M, Ishida S. Impaired circulation in the thickened choroid of a patient with serpiginous choroiditis. Ocul Immunol Inflamm. 2014; 22(5):409–413

[37] D'Ambrosio E, Tortorella P, Iannetti L. Management of uveitis-related choroidal neovascularization: from the pathogenesis to the therapy. J Ophthalmol. 2014; 2014:450428

[38] Parodi MB, Iacono P, La Spina C, et al. Intravitreal bevacizumab for choroidal neovascularisation in serpiginous choroiditis. Br J Ophthalmol. 2014; 98(4):519–522

[39] Kuehlewein L, Bansal M, Lenis TL, et al. Optical coherence tomography angiography of type 1 neovascularization in age-related macular degeneration. Am J Ophthalmol. 2015; 160(4):739–48.e2

[40] Baumal CR, de Carlo TE, Waheed NK, Salz DA, Witkin AJ, Duker JS. Sequential optical coherence tomographic angiography for diagnosis and treatment of choroidal neovascularization in multifocal choroiditis. JAMA Ophthalmol. 2015; 133(9):1087–1090

[41] Costanzo E, Cohen SY, Miere A, et al. Optical coherence tomography angiography in central serous chorior-etinopathy. J Ophthalmol. 2015; 2015:134783

15 Optical Coherence Tomography Angiography Findings in Ocular Oncology and Radiation Retinopathy

Meghna V. Motiani, Colin A. McCannel, and Tara A. McCannel

Summary

The use of optical coherence tomography angiography (OCTA) in ocular oncology is currently in its infancy. However, the ability of OCTA to significantly improve the evaluation of the retinal vasculature may have its greatest application in the evaluation and management of radiation retinopathy. Here, we provide an overview of the role of OCTA in the setting of ophthalmic tumors and radiation retinopathy. A series of examples of OCTA images associated with common intraocular tumors is presented.

Keywords: OCTA, optical coherence tomography angiography, intraocular tumor, uveal melanoma, radiation retinopathy

15.1 Introduction

Intraocular tumors comprise a spectrum of benign and malignant entities, from the choroid to the retina. Conventional ocular imaging techniques, such as color photography, fluorescein angiography, ultrasonography and optical coherence tomography (OCT) have been important tools for use alongside the clinical examination in diagnosing ocular tumors and in monitoring their response to treatment.[1]

Radiation therapy is the most common method to treat malignant intraocular tumors of the eye. However, although highly successful at limiting tumor growth, radiation retinopathy often results in irreparable visual loss from vascular damage at the macula and elsewhere in the fundus. Previous reports suggest that almost half of patients who undergo brachytherapy for local tumor control of choroidal melanoma may have vision worse than 20/200 in 3 years.[2] Multimodal imaging techniques, including OCT and wide-field fluorescein angiography, may help detect radiation retinopathy before the visual acuity is affected.

The management of radiation retinopathy continues to evolve. Although intravitreal anti–vascular endothelial growth factor (anti-VEGF) or steroids may be given to treat macular edema, long-term beneficial results are lacking. Furthermore, the benefit of early treatment of radiation retinopathy has not been clearly established. Post-radiation treatment of retinal ischemia and proliferative retinopathy may likely benefit from pan retinal laser photocoagulation to prevent vitreous hemorrhage, neovascular glaucoma, and a cascade of events leading to a "blind painful eye" requiring enucleation. Reducing the radiation exposure to healthy nontumor tissue with silicone oil 1,000 centistokes as a vitreous substitute during brachytherapy has been demonstrated to reduce radiation retinopathy and improve visual acuity.[3,4,5]

Despite treatment controversy, new imaging modalities to identify the effects of radiation on the retinal vasculature may enhance our understanding of the disease. Furthermore, defining quantitative parameters to localize radiation retinopathy may be useful when evaluating novel techniques to prevent or treat this entity in patients.

OCT angiography (OCTA) is a novel noninvasive imaging modality that utilizes motion contrast of blood flow to generate a series of angiographic images.[6,7] It enables exquisite visualization of each layer of the retina in a continuous, three-dimensional fashion.[6,7,8] Moreover, software algorithms can calculate the foveal avascular zone and capillary vascular density. As such, a numeric value can be assigned to the level of pathology, in contrast to the qualitative descriptions to which we are accustomed in clinical ophthalmology.

In addition to the retina, the choriocapillaris and choroidal layers may also be evaluated with OCTA. Unlike the retina, where vascular patterns and details are readily discernable, images of the choroid may be more variable and ill defined, and are known to vary in appearance between different OCTA platforms. Because most intraocular tumors originate from the choroid, this presents a challenge in the OCTA description of tumors, and may explain why most published reports on OCTA feature analysis of the retinal layers rather than the choroidal layers. However, with continued evolution of OCTA and anticipated improvements in visualization of choroidal details, one can expect that primary intraocular tumor evaluation with OCTA holds promise.

The application of OCTA for the evaluation of common ophthalmologic diseases such as age-related macular degeneration, diabetic retinopathy, retinal vascular disease, and glaucoma has been described in the literature and in more detail elsewhere in this book.[6,7,9,10,11,12] However, there are few reports describing OCTA findings in the context of ocular oncology. The purpose of this chapter is to describe the typical OCTA findings associated with intraocular tumors and radiation retinopathy. We have chosen to present images in three planes: (1) superficial retina, (2) deep retina, and (3) choriocapillaris and/or choroid.

15.2 Posterior Segment Tumors

15.2.1 Retinal Tumors

Melanocytoma

Melanocytoma is most frequently observed at the optic disc more often in pigmented individuals, although these lesions may sometimes involve the choroid or iris. Unlike in choroidal nevus or choroidal melanoma, the typical optic disc melanocytoma infiltrates the retina, and retinal disorganization may be observed with spectral-domain OCT (SD-OCT).[13,14]

Although there have been no previously published reports on OCTA findings in optic disc melanocytoma, we have observed findings that are similar to established OCT findings. Vascular tortuosity with increased capillary volume density is observed at the superficial retinal layer (▶ Fig. 15.1). Both the deep retinal vascular layer and the choriocapillaris layer feature prominent signal void at the site of the lesion, which may

arise from vascular signal blockage associated with the pigmented cells of the lesion. It is clear from OCTA that posterior melanocytomas are characterized by features that are distinct from both choroidal nevi and choroidal melanomas, where in these latter lesions there is usually no superficial retinal vascular alteration (see sections "Choroidal Nevus" and "Choroidal Melanoma").

15.2.2 Retinal Pigment Epithelial Tumors

Tumors of the retinal pigment epithelium (RPE) are most commonly represented by the benign congenital hypertrophy of the retinal pigment epithelial lesion. However, retinal pigment epithelial adenomas, most commonly found in the retinal periphery and retinal pigment epithelial adenocarcinomas, also comprise this group of tumors.

Congenital Hypertrophy of the Retinal Pigment Epithelium

Congenital hypertrophy of the retinal pigment epithelium (CHRPE) is a fairly common peripheral benign tumor of the RPE that has well-defined borders and may contain lacunae, or areas of depigmentation. These tumors rarely undergo malignant transformation. Occasionally, in young pigmented individuals with myopia, these benign tumors may simulate the appearance of an elevated choroidal mass and be mistaken for a choroidal melanoma.[15]

As most CHRPE lesions are located in the retinal periphery, they may be difficult to characterize by OCTA. We have found that the superficial and deep

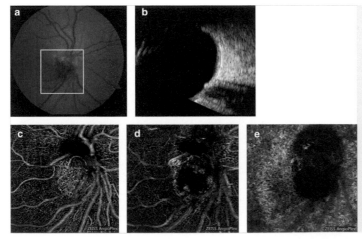

Fig. 15.1 Melanocytoma.
(a) Peripapillary melanocytoma.
(b) A 1.1-mm height by B-scan.
(c) Superficial retina optical coherence tomography angiography (OCTA) reveals discrete cluster of irregular overlying vessels, which appear to be dilated and distorted superficial retinal capillaries. Deep retina OCTA
(d) reveals central signal void, presumably from pigment signal blockage. Similarly, the choriocapillaris OCTA (e) layer reveals signal void in the area of the lesion.

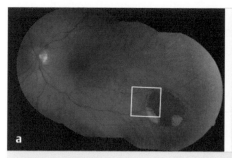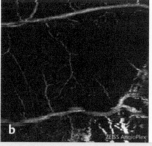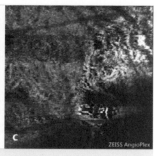

Fig. 15.2 Congenital hypertrophy of the retinal pigment epithelium. (a) Discrete flat inferotemporal tumor with inferior lacunae. (b) Superficial retina optical coherence tomography angiography (OCTA) reveals minimal vascular abnormality. (c) Choriocapillaris OCTA shows some hyper-reflectivity and central signal void likely corresponding to lesion hyperpigmentation.

retinal layers are minimally altered. However, the choriocapillaris and choroidal layers clearly demonstrate the borders of the lesion and show signal void associated with the lesion with greater penetration to the choroid (▶ Fig. 15.2).

15.2.3 Choroidal Tumors

Determining distinguishing features of macular choroidal lesions on OCTA has been somewhat challenging because OCTA may not be the ideal tool for evaluating choroidal vasculature, and rarely do the superficial retinal vessels overlying a choroidal mass display any clinically abnormal features. Furthermore, lesions that are elevated and greater than 2.0 mm result in areas of flow-void and present challenges with optical capture.

Choroidal Nevus

Choroidal nevi are the most common intraocular tumors, with a higher prevalence among Caucasians (0.2 to 20%) compared to other races.[14,16] They do not often cause visual symptoms, and on examination are typically pigmented with smooth margins and may have overlying drusen. Although choroidal nevi are benign, it has been estimated that 1 in 8,845 choroidal nevi undergoes transformation to choroidal melanoma.[14] As such, careful evaluation and follow-up is advised, particularly in elevated choroidal nevi.

OCT has been used to differentiate nevi from melanomas, and also to identify features that predict transformation. Overlying drusen are found in 40% of choroidal nevi, and manifest as small, dome-shaped elevations at the level of the RPE/ Bruch's membrane.[14] Other common imaging

features on OCT include choroidal shadowing deep to the nevus, choriocapillaris thinning overlying the nevus, RPE atrophy or loss, RPE modularity, photoreceptor loss, ellipsoid zone irregularity or loss, external limiting membrane irregularity, outer nuclear and outer plexiform layer irregularity, inner nuclear layer irregularity, and subretinal fluid.[16]

OCT has a higher sensitivity than clinical examination in the detection and characterization of overlying intraretinal edema, subretinal fluid, retinal atrophy, and RPE detachment. These features are significant, and may influence foveal vision in macular nevi, as well as represent features of malignant transformation.[14]

Valverde-Megías et al reported on the OCTA findings of central macular thickness, superficial and deep foveal avascular zone, and capillary vascular density of the macula in 70 eyes harboring a nevus outside the macula (average thickness: 1.38 mm; range: 0–2.4 mm) compared to the macular findings in the contralateral eye. There were no significant differences in these parameters of the macula between the normal and the nevus eye.[17]

The OCTA features through a flat choroidal nevus are depicted in ▶ Fig. 15.3 and ▶ Fig. 15.4, and an elevated choroidal nevus in ▶ Fig. 15.5 and ▶ Fig. 15.6. As previously reported, choroidal nevi do not generally result in alteration of the overlying retinal vasculature. However, as the thickness of the lesion increases, the elevation through the deep retinal layers may manifest as signal void. Given the origin of these lesions in the choroidal layer, choroidal nevi demonstrate most of the OCTA alterations in the choriocapillaris and deep choroidal layers. At the more superficial choriocapillaris, signal void is observed at the site of the

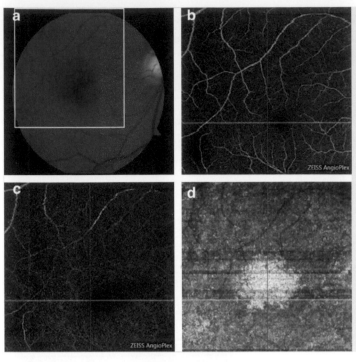

Fig. 15.3 Choroidal nevus. **(a)** Flat macular choroidal nevus. **(b)** Superficial retina optical coherence tomography angiography (OCTA) reveals no apparent vascular abnormality. **(c)** Deep retina OCTA reveals slightly irregular vessels over the lesion. **(d)** Choriocapillaris and deeper choroidal layers reveal hyper-reflective area corresponding to the pigmented choroidal lesion, without clear visible changes in the choriocapillaris.

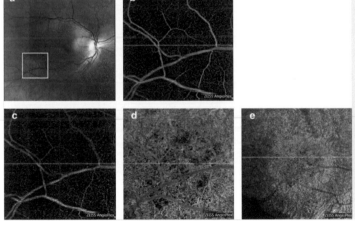

Fig. 15.4 Choroidal nevus. **(a)** Flat macular choroidal nevus. **(b)** Superficial retina optical coherence tomography angiography (OCTA) reveals no apparent vascular abnormality. **(c)** Deep retina OCTA reveals no abnormality. **(d)** Choriocapillaris reveals signal void corresponding to nevus, and **(e)** deeper choroid OCTA reveals hyper-reflective area corresponding to lesion with areas of relative hyporeflective change corresponding to areas of hypopigmentation of the lesion.

choroidal nevus. In the deeper choroidal layer, hyper-reflectivity may be observed. The etiology of the hyper-reflectivity is not clearly understood, but may represent the density of the choroidal pigment, which comprises these lesions.

Choroidal Melanoma

Uveal melanoma is the most common primary intraocular malignancy in adults, and 90% develop in the choroid.[14] The focus of this section will be on posterior uveal melanoma, otherwise described as choroidal melanoma. Clinical examination reveals an elevated choroidal mass sometimes with serous retinal detachment. Multimodal imaging identifies features of activity and leakage.

Relatively little is known about the OCTA findings associated with choroidal melanoma. Previous evaluation of macular OCTA findings, regardless of location of the actual tumor, has revealed an enlargement of the deep foveal avascular zone and a reduction in superficial and deep capillary

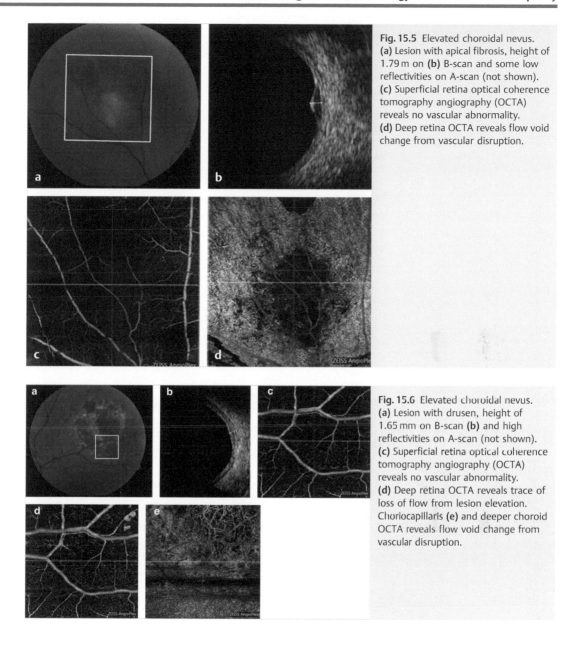

Fig. 15.5 Elevated choroidal nevus. **(a)** Lesion with apical fibrosis, height of 1.79 m on **(b)** B-scan and some low reflectivities on A-scan (not shown). **(c)** Superficial retina optical coherence tomography angiography (OCTA) reveals no vascular abnormality. **(d)** Deep retina OCTA reveals flow void change from vascular disruption.

Fig. 15.6 Elevated choroidal nevus. **(a)** Lesion with drusen, height of 1.65 mm on B-scan **(b)** and high reflectivities on A-scan (not shown). **(c)** Superficial retina optical coherence tomography angiography (OCTA) reveals no vascular abnormality. **(d)** Deep retina OCTA reveals trace of loss of flow from lesion elevation. Choriocapillaris **(e)** and deeper choroid OCTA reveals flow void change from vascular disruption.

vascular density. The extent of these vascular alterations were dependent on tumor size, suggesting that parafoveal microvascular ischemia was caused by the melanomas themselves.[17,18]

OCTA through the melanoma itself may be most useful in the evaluation of small uveal melanoma (i.e., <2.0 mm) as there is less choroidal elevation to alter the superficial and deep retinal layers. Examples of small choroidal melanoma and their corresponding OCTA images are demonstrated in ▶ Fig. 15.7 and ▶ Fig. 15.8. In tumors of thickness

less than 2.0 mm, there is often no significant vascular alteration in the superficial retinal layer. The deep retinal layer may demonstrate mild to moderate loss of vessels overlying the tumor. The choroid layer may reveal mostly loss of signal in the area of the melanoma.

Choroidal Metastasis

Choroidal metastatic tumors are the most common intraocular neoplasm of adults. Without a

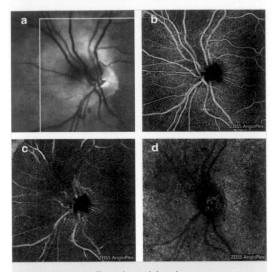

Fig. 15.7 Peripapillary choroidal melanoma.
(a) Peripapillary elevated melanoma with pigmentation.
(b) Superficial retina optical coherence tomography angiography (OCTA) reveals minimal vascular abnormality. **(c)** Deep retina OCTA reveals mild loss of vessels overlying lesion. **(d)** Choriocapillaris OCTA shows trace of flow void at apex of lesion, most pronounced at lesion hyperpigmentation.

known medical history of cancer, however, making the diagnosis of metastatic tumor may be challenging. The vast majority of ocular metastatic tumors develop in the choroid perhaps because of its rich vascular supply.[1,14] Well-described clinical features, such as yellow coloration, irregular borders, multiple lesions, bilateral involvement, and irregular appearance on ultrasonography may assist in making the correct clinical diagnosis. Most patients have a prior history of systemic cancer: breast cancer is the most common type to

metastasize, accounting for 48 to 53% of cases.[14] This is followed by prostate cancer, cutaneous melanoma, and lung cancer.[1,16] Among the 34% of patients who do not have a history of cancer, the lung is the most common primary source after evaluation.[14]

There have been no previous reports of OCTA findings regarding choroidal metastatic tumors. Findings may be somewhat similar to choroidal melanoma, a sometimes-similar appearing malignant neoplasm of the choroid. As such, we have found choroidal metastatic tumors to have minimal alteration of the superficial retinal layer, mild alteration of the deep retinal layer, and signal void in the choroidal layer (▶ Fig. 15.9).

Choroidal Hemangioma

Choroidal hemangiomas are benign vascular tumors that assume a circumscribed or diffuse pattern, based on the extent of choroidal involvement.[14] Diagnosis can be challenging: on funduscopy, they may resemble other melanotic choroidal lesions such as choroidal melanoma, choroidal metastases, posterior scleritis, choroidal granuloma, choroidal osteoma, lymphoma, or atypical central serous retinopathy.[16] Circumscribed hemangiomas are usually orange colored, round, and located in the posterior pole, near the optic disc.[14,19] Diffuse hemangiomas, by contrast, usually extend to involve the entire choroid and are often associated with ipsilateral facial hemangiomas in the context of the Sturge–Weber syndrome.[14]

Although ultrasound and indocyanine green (ICG) are traditionally most helpful in the diagnosis of these lesions, OCT can be used to evaluate secondary retinal morphologic changes.[19] In

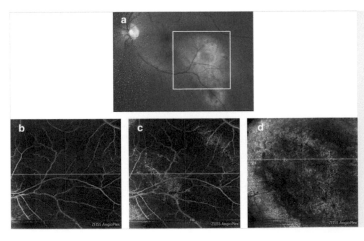

Fig. 15.8 Choroidal melanoma.
(a) Parafoveal melanoma, height of 2.3 mm. **(b)** Superficial retina optical coherence tomography angiography (OCTA) reveals mild vascular disruption. **(c)** Deep retina OCTA reveals moderate loss of vessels overlying and adjacent to lesion. **(d)** Choriocapillaris OCTA shows flow void at lesion, maximal at center.

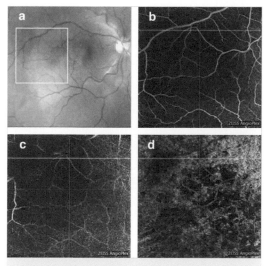

Fig. 15.9 Choroidal metastasis. **(a)** Yellow lesion with ill-defined borders in temporal macula, in patient with primary lung adenocarcinoma. **(b)** Superficial retina optical coherence tomography angiography (OCTA) reveals no vascular disturbance. **(c)** Deep retina OCTA reveals some loss of flow at tumor. **(d)** Choriocapillaris OCTA reveals signal void corresponding to lesion.

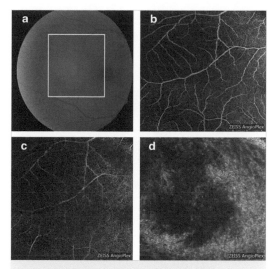

Fig. 15.10 Choroidal hemangioma. **(a)** Orange-colored dome-shaped choroidal tumor of macula. **(b)** Superficial retina optical coherence tomography angiography (OCTA) reveals no significant vessel alteration. **(c)** Deep retina OCTA reveals mild loss of vessels overlying lesion. **(d)** Choriocapillaris OCTA demonstrates uniform central signal void at center of lesion.

patients with the circumscribed variant, characteristic features include subretinal fluid (10%), retinal edema (42%), retinal schisms (12%), macular edema (24%), and localized photoreceptor loss (35%).[16,19] Patients with the diffuse variant often display subretinal fluid (28%), retinal edema (14%), and photoreceptor loss (43%).[16]

There have been no previous reports of OCTA findings to date associated with choroidal hemangioma. Similar to other choroidal tumors (such as melanoma or metastasis), choroidal hemangiomas demonstrate minimal alteration of the superficial retinal layer, mild alteration of the deep retinal layer, and signal void in the choroidal layer (▶ Fig. 15.10).

Choroidal Osteoma

Choroidal osteomas are rare, osseous tumors often found in young females. They are benign, but have the capacity to grow: long-term studies show growth rates of 41 to 51%.[14] On clinical examination, these lesions appear as an orange-yellow plaque in the juxtapapillary region or macula, and can demonstrate areas of whitening when decalcified.

The internal structure of choroidal osteomas is difficult to evaluate with OCT, and is limited to its anterior surface and resultant changes of the

overlying retina. Heterogeneity of these tumors depends on the amount of calcification. Calcified portions of the tumor reveal intact inner and outer retinal layers, a distinct RPE, and mild transmission of light. Decalcified portions of the tumor, by contrast, reveal intact inner retinal layers, thinned outer retinal layers, an indistinct RPE, and marked light transmission into the tumor.

Features of choroidal osteoma themselves have not been well characterized by OCTA. We have found that there is minimal to no alteration of the superficial and deep retinal layers and the choroidal layer reveals signal loss associated with the lesion (▶ Fig. 15.11 and ▶ Fig. 15.12). The location of the osteoma, whether diffusely in the macula or focal extramacula, does not seem to influence these features.

Choroidal neovascularization may be a potentially sight-threatening complication associated with choroidal osteoma, particularly when the macula is involved. Anti-VEGF agents may be promptly instituted if this complication is detected. Szelog et al reported the use of OCTA to identify the vascular complex of neovascularization that was not identifiable by standard fluorescein angiography.[20]

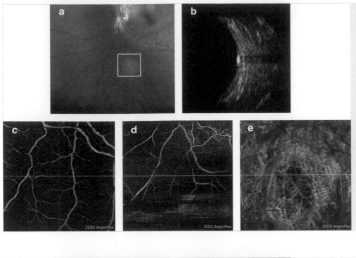

Fig. 15.11 Choroidal osteoma.
(a) Discrete amelanotic plaquelike choroidal lesion with shadowing from calcification on **(b)** B-scan.
(c) Superficial retina optical coherence tomography angiography (OCTA) reveals no vascular abnormality.
(d) Deep retina OCTA reveals normal vasculature. Choriocapillaris and **(e)** deeper choroid OCTA reveals flow void alteration from vascular disruption at center of lesion.

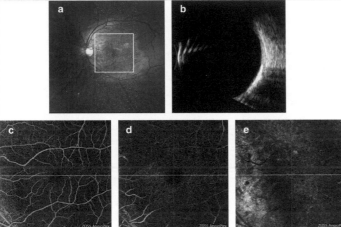

Fig. 15.12 Choroidal osteoma.
(a) Extensive macula-involving discrete choroidal tumor with orbital shadowing on **(b)** B-scan.
(c) Superficial retina optical coherence tomography angiography (OCTA) reveals no vascular abnormality.
(d) Deep retina OCTA reveals diffuse loss of vessels at center of lesion.
(e) Choriocapillaris OCTA shows irregular hyper-reflective areas.

Idiopathic Scleral Choroidal Calcification

Scleral choroidal calcification is the result of calcium salts in the sclera and choroid, which is usually idiopathic, but has been reported to be associated with hypercalcemia or rare systemic syndromes. This lesion is usually bilateral and found in the superotemporal quadrants. The lesion may consist of multiple discrete yellow placoid lesions.

OCTA of scleral choroidal calcification reveals discrete areas of hyper-reflectivity in both the superficial and deep retinal layers that correspond to the actual yellow placoid lesions themselves. In the choroidal layer, there is dramatic signal loss corresponding to the lesions (▸ Fig. 15.13).

Although the ultrasonographic features of both scleral choroidal calcification and choroidal osteoma may be indistinguishable, clearly the OCTA features of idiopathic scleral choroidal calcification appear to involve all levels of the retina on OCTA imaging.

15.3 Cancer Associated Ocular Vascular Complications

15.3.1 Radiation Treatment of Choroidal Tumors

Radiation therapy can be used to achieve local tumor control for choroidal melanomas and choroidal metastases. Following therapy, successful treatment occurs when there is no further growth of the tumor. Although primary choroidal melanoma requires a higher radiation dose to achieve

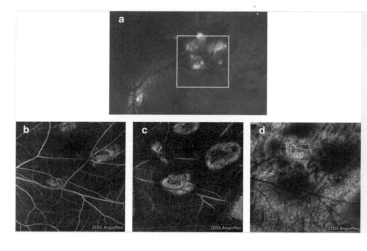

Fig. 15.13 Scleral choroidal calcification. **(a)** Discrete superotemporal areas of placoid choroidal calcification. **(b)** Superficial retina optical coherence tomography angiography (OCTA) reveals hyper-reflective areas at the tumor. **(c)** Deep retina OCTA reveals further emphasis of focal areas. **(d)** Choriocapillaris OCTA demonstrates contrasting signal void at respective areas of lesion.

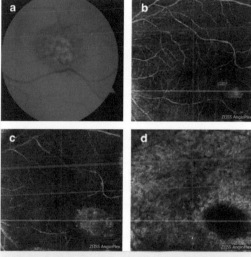

Fig. 15.14 Treated small choroidal melanoma. **(a)** Choroidal melanoma status post-iodine-125 brachytherapy 3 months ago. **(b)** Superficial retina optical coherence tomography angiography (OCTA) reveals hyper-reflectivity at tumor surface. **(c)** Deep retina OCTA reveals increased hyper-reflectivity. **(d)** Choriocapillaris OCTA demonstrates discrete flow void at center of melanoma.

local control than metastatic tumors, both tumors can be successfully treated with brachytherapy. Multimodal imaging of treated choroidal melanoma or choroidal metastatic tumor results in atrophy associated with the overlying retina, loss of pigmentation, and generalized chorioretinal atrophy in the bed of the radiation plaque.

OCTA findings associated with a treated choroidal tumor are variable and generally depend on the length of time that the tumor was treated. Choroidal melanoma that has recently been treated may demonstrate very little clinical change compared to a melanoma that was treated over 5 years previously, when significant atrophy associated with the tumor may be observed.

▶ Fig. 15.14 demonstrates the OCTA appearance of a 1.79-mm-thick choroidal melanoma 3 months following iodine-125 brachytherapy. There is little overlying change of the superficial or deep retina. However, the choroidal layer demonstrates pruning of vessels at the margins of the tumor and signal loss central to the tumor. Untreated melanomas typically show signal loss at the choroidal layer; however, the pruned appearance of the choroidal vessels may be more characteristic of a treated tumor. ▶ Fig. 15.15 demonstrates the OCTA appearance of a 1.50-mm-thick melanoma 3 months after brachytherapy. Both the superficial and deep layers reveal the prominent lipofuscin of the tumor, with little other vascular change; the deeper choroidal layer demonstrates signal loss with slight pruning effect at the tumor margins. ▶ Fig. 15.16 demonstrates the OCTA appearance of a 1.70-mm-thick melanoma 2 years following brachytherapy. There is capillary vascular density loss particularly in the temporal macular of the superficial and deep retinal layers; however, there is prominent signal loss and pruning effect of the choroidal vessels at the treated tumor. We have observed that the choroidal pruning appearance and signal loss become more pronounced with time from treatment.

▶ Fig. 15.17 demonstrates the appearance of a treated choroidal metastatic tumor 2 years following iodine-125 brachytherapy. There is some mild alteration in the overlying superficial and deep

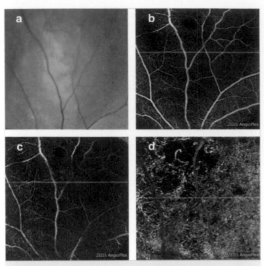

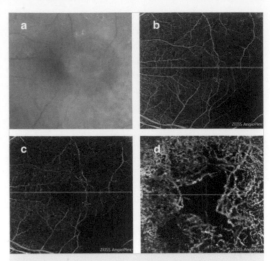

Fig. 15.15 Treated small choroidal melanoma. **(a)** Choroidal melanoma status post-iodine-125 brachytherapy 3 months ago. **(b)** Superficial retina optical coherence tomography angiography (OCTA) reveals normal vessels. **(c)** Deep retina OCTA reveals mild disruption of vessels. **(d)** Choriocapillaris OCTA shows vascular loss and pruning of vessels surrounding tumor.

Fig. 15.16 Treated small macular choroidal melanoma. **(a)** Macular choroidal melanoma status post-iodine-125 brachytherapy 2 years ago. **(b)** Superficial retina optical coherence tomography angiography (OCTA) reveals altered overlying vessels. **(c)** Deep retina OCTA reveals more prominent disruption of vessels. **(d)** Choriocapillaris OCTA shows signal void at the central aspect of tumor, with pruning of vessels surrounding tumor.

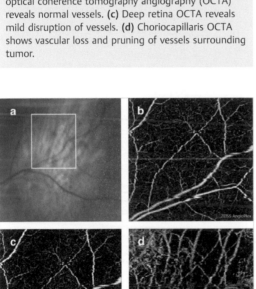

Fig. 15.17 Treated choroidal metastatic tumor. **(a)** Flat chorioretinal atrophy following brachytherapy 2 years ago for choroidal metastatic tumor in patient with primary non–small cell lung carcinoma. **(b)** Superficial retina optical coherence tomography angiography (OCTA) reveals minimal alteration. **(c)** Deep retina OCTA reveals mild loss of vessels overlying lesion. **(d)** Choriocapillaris OCTA shows reduction of vascularity at site of lesion.

retinal vascular layers, and signal loss of the choroid layer (although some vessels still persist).

15.3.2 Radiation Retinopathy

Radiation retinopathy is the leading cause of visual loss in patients who have undergone radiotherapy for local tumor control. The range of retinopathy includes macular edema and may progress to panfundus retinal ischemia, which may include a propensity for proliferative radiation.[21] Clinically, radiation maculopathy may include retinal hemorrhages and cotton wool spots. However, OCT has allowed for early detection of capillary damage often before the patient is clinically symptomatic.

Recently, in a description of seven cases of radiation retinopathy, Veverka et al demonstrated that OCTA of the deep and superficial retinal vasculature may reveal a widened foveal avascular zone and capillary dropout prior to the development of retinal edema or defect on conventional OCT imaging through the macula.[22]

Say et al also noted this finding: among 10 eyes treated with iodine-125 brachytherapy, there was a decrease in capillary vascular density compared to their untreated fellow eye. All patients had clinically normal findings, otherwise. The authors postulate that this is the earliest manifestation of radiation retinopathy.[23]

▶ Fig. 15.18 demonstrates macular findings associated with a posteriorly located choroidal melanoma treated with combined iodine-125 brachytherapy and vitrectomy with silicone oil for radiation attenuation 2 years previously. Although the visual acuity is 20/20 and the SD-OCT appears normal, there are multiple focal areas of capillary vascular dropout in both superficial and deep retinal layers of the treated eye compared to the normal OCTA of the fellow eye.

Enlargement of the foveal avascular zone and reduction in capillary vascular density may be expected with progression of radiation maculopathy. ▶ Fig. 15.19 demonstrates macular findings

associated with a choroidal melanoma treated with iodine-125 brachytherapy 9 years previously with 20/400 vision. The SD-OCT reveals exudates, retinal edema, and atrophy. With this more advanced level of radiation maculopathy, there is further enlargement of the foveal avascular zone and reduction in capillary vascular density in the treated eye at both superficial and deep retinal vascular layers.

▶ Fig. 15.20 demonstrates the macular findings associated with a choroidal melanoma treated with iodine-125 brachytherapy 8 years previously, but with worse vision at counting fingers. The OCT reveals cystic edema and diffuse macular atrophy. Further reduction in capillary vascular density and vascular irregularities are observed in both the superficial and the deep retinal vascular layers.

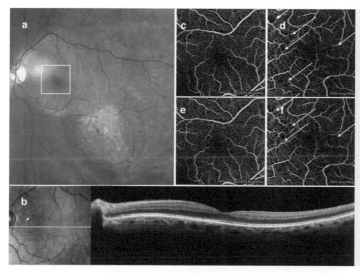

Fig. 15.18 Early radiation maculopathy. **(a)** Choroidal melanoma treated 2 years ago with iodine-125 and silicone oil for radiation attenuation with 20/20 vision and normal retinal contour on **(b)** spectral-domain optical coherence tomography (SD-OCT) B-scan. Compared to the **(c)** normal fellow eye, superficial **(d)** retina OCT angiography (OCTA) reveals mild loss in capillary density with perifoveal areas of flow void (arrows). compared to the **(e)** normal eye, **(f)** Deep retina OCTA reveals similar flow void areas (arrows).

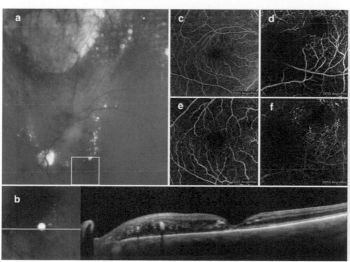

Fig. 15.19 Moderate radiation maculopathy. **(a)** Choroidal melanoma treated 9 years ago with iodine-125 brachytherapy, with 20/400 vision. **(b)** Spectral-domain optical coherence tomography (SD-OCT) B-scan shows abnormal retinal contour, intraretinal hyper-reflective material (exudate), intraretinal edema, and foveal atrophy. Compared to the **(c)** normal fellow eye, **(d)** superficial retina OCT angiography (OCTA) reveals enlarged foveal avascular zone and significant loss in capillary vascular density. Compared to the **(e)** normal fellow eye, **(f)** deep retina OCTA reveals similar findings.

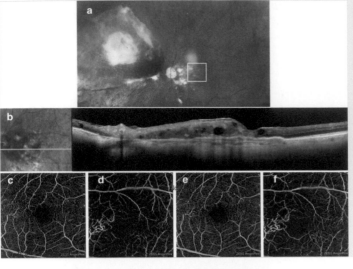

Fig. 15.20 Advanced radiation maculopathy. **(a)** Choroidal melanoma treated 8 years ago with iodine-125 brachytherapy, with counting fingers vision. **(b)** Spectral-domain optical coherence tomography (SD-OCT) B-scan shows diffuse macular atrophy and intraretinal edema. Compared to the **(c)** normal fellow eye, **(d)** superficial retina OCT angiography (OCTA) reveals severe loss in capillary vascular density with enlarged foveal avascular zone. Compared to the **(e)** normal fellow eye, **(f)** deep retina OCTA reveals similar findings.

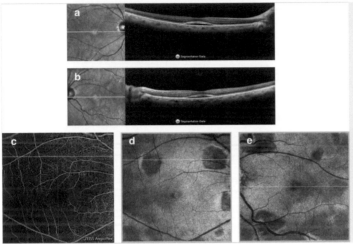

Fig. 15.21 MEK-inhibitor maculopathy spectral-domain optical coherence tomography (SD-OCT) reveals subfoveal serous detachment of the retina in **(a)** right and **(b)** left macula; red-free reveals mostly foveal irregularity. **(c)** Superficial retina OCT angiography (OCTA) reveals little vascular disruption. **(d)** En face analysis of the right eye identifies multiple focal retinal detachments more prominent than clinical examination or standard SD-OCT. **(e)** En face analysis of left eye showing similar multiple areas of focal retinal detachment.

15.4 MEK-Inhibitor Maculopathy

A new class of mitogen-activated protein kinase (MAP-kinase) associated inhibitors, which block cancer proliferation, was recently approved for the treatment of metastatic cancers.[24] These agents have been associated with single or multiple macular serous retinal detachments, which are dose-dependent and generally self-limited.[25,26,27] Although difficult to detect on clinical examination, OCT has been fairly sensitive in detecting these mostly subclinical findings. We have found that OCTA, however, is even more sensitive at detecting these lesions, particularly with the en face imaging feature.

▶ Fig. 15.21 demonstrates both the bilateral SD-OCT features and the increase in number of lesions detectable with en face OCT imaging.

15.5 Conclusion

There are limitations of OCTA in ocular oncology. Some of the challenges include the difficulty of segmenting the capillary layers in the retina overlying tumors due to the dome-shaped or irregular contour of a tumor surface. This is particularly true for tumors of increasing height. As a result, there is often signal void with a rim of vasculature and capillary visibility. The heavy pigmentation of many lesions seen in the fundus (including nevi, melanomas, and melanocytomas) can introduce challenges of signal absorption, or in some cases high signal reflectivity. Moreover, it is difficult to image lesions beyond the macula, which may also limit the utility of OCTA for many lesions. However, future technologic advances may overcome this shortcoming. Furthermore, assessment of the peripheral retina, where significant radiation retinopathy occurs, will continue to demand the use of fluorescein angiography (and in particular wide-field imaging) for thorough evaluation, due to the limitations of OCTA beyond the macular region.

The ability of OCTA to provide great detail of even subtle retinal vascular changes promises to allow further characterization of the retinal vascular damage induced by ocular tumors themselves and their treatment. Most notably, OCTA will likely facilitate more careful study of radiation retinopathy, its prevention, and treatment. The ability to quantitate the macular vasculature will be a valuable tool in evaluating treatment interventions and outcomes.

References

[1] Tailor TD, Gupta D, Dalley RW, Keene CD, Anzai Y. Orbital neoplasms in adults: clinical, radiologic, and pathologic review. Radiographics. 2013; 33(6):1739–1758

[2] Melia BM, Abramson DH, Albert DM, et al. Collaborative Ocular Melanoma Study Group. Collaborative ocular melanoma study (COMS) randomized trial of I-125 brachytherapy for medium choroidal melanoma. I. Visual acuity after 3 years COMS report no. 16. Ophthalmology. 2001; 108(2):348–366

[3] Oliver SC, Leu MY, DeMarco JJ, Chow PE, Lee SP, McCannel TA. Attenuation of iodine 125 radiation with vitreous substitutes in the treatment of uveal melanoma. Arch Ophthalmol. 2010; 128(7):888–893

[4] McCannel TA, McCannel CA. Iodine 125 brachytherapy with vitrectomy and silicone oil in the treatment of uveal melanoma: 1-to-1 matched case-control series. Int J Radiat Oncol Biol Phys. 2014; 89(2):347–352

[5] McCannel TA, Kamrava M, Demanes J, et al. 23-mm iodine-125 plaque for uveal melanoma: benefit of vitrectomy and silicone oil on visual acuity. Graefes Arch Clin Exp Ophthalmol. 2016; 254(12):2461–2467

[6] Chalam KV, Sambhav K. Optical coherence tomography angiography in retinal diseases. J Ophthalmic Vis Res. 2016; 11(1):84–92

[7] de Carlo TE, Romano A, Waheed NK, Duker JS. A review of optical coherence tomography angiography (OCTA). Int J Retina Vitreous. 2015; 1(5):5

[8] Choi W, Mohler KJ, Potsaid B, et al. Choriocapillaris and choroidal microvasculature imaging with ultrahigh speed OCT angiography. PLoS One. 2013; 8(12):e81499

[9] Fang PP, Lindner M, Steinberg JS, et al. Clinical applications of OCT angiography. Ophthalmologe. 2016; 113(1):14–22

[10] Liu L, Jia Y, Takusagawa HL, et al. Optical coherence tomography angiography of the peripapillary retina in glaucoma. JAMA Ophthalmol. 2015; 133(9):1045–1052

[11] Ishibazawa A, Nagaoka T, Takahashi A, et al. Optical coherence tomography angiography in diabetic retinopathy: a prospective pilot study. Am J Ophthalmol. 2015; 160(1):35–44.e1

[12] Freiberg FJ, Pfau M, Wons J, Wirth MA, Becker MD, Michels S. Optical coherence tomography angiography of the foveal avascular zone in diabetic retinopathy. Graefes Arch Clin Exp Ophthalmol. 2016; 254(6):1051–1058

[13] Shields CL, Kaliki S, Rojanaporn D, Ferenczy SR, Shields JA. Enhanced depth imaging optical coherence tomography of small choroidal melanoma: comparison with choroidal nevus. Arch Ophthalmol. 2012; 130(7):850–856

[14] Say EAT, Shah SU, Ferenczy S, Shields CL. Optical coherence tomography of retinal and choroidal tumors. J Ophthalmol. 2011; 2011–385058

[15] Chang MY, McBeath JB, McCannel CA, McCannel TA. "Shadow sign" in congenital hypertrophy of the retinal pigment epithelium of young myopic pigmented patients. Eye (Lond). 2016; 30(1):160–163

[16] Medina CA, Plesec T, Singh AD. Optical coherence tomography imaging of ocular and periocular tumours. Br J Ophthalmol. 2014; 98 Suppl 2:ii40–ii46

[17] Verdes-Malva A, Say EA, Ferenczy SR, Shields CL. Differential macular features on optical coherence tomography angiography in eyes with choroidal nevus and melanoma. Retina. 2017; 37(4):731–740

[18] Li Y, Say EA, Ferenczy S, Agni M, Shields CL. Altered parafoveal microvasculature in treatment-naive choroidal melanoma eyes detected by optical coherence tomography angiography. Retina. 2017; 37(1):32–40

[19] Heimann H, Jmor F, Damato B. Imaging of retinal and choroidal vascular tumours. Eye (Lond). 2013; 27(2):208–216

[20] Szelog JT, Bonini Filho MA, Lally DR, de Carlo TE, Duker JS. Optical coherence tomography angiography for detecting choroidal neovascularization secondary to choroidal osteoma. Ophthalmic Surg Lasers Imaging Retina. 2016; 47(1):69–72

[21] Wen JC, Oliver SC, McCannel TA. Ocular complications following I-125 brachytherapy for choroidal melanoma. Eye (Lond). 2009; 23(6):1254–1268

[22] Veverka KK, AbouChehade JE, Iezzi R, Jr, Pulido JS. Noninvasive grading of radiation retinopathy: the use of optical coherence tomography angiography. Retina. 2015; 35(11):2400–2410

[23] Say EA, Samara WA, Khoo CT, et al. Parafoveal capillary density after plaque radiotherapy for choroidal melanoma: analysis of eyes without radiation maculopathy. Retina. 2016; 36(9):1670–1678

[24] Flaherty KT, Robert C, Hersey P, et al. METRIC Study Group. Improved survival with MEK inhibition in BRAF-mutated melanoma. N Engl J Med. 2012; 367(2):107–114

[25] McCannel TA, Chmielowski B, Finn RS, et al. Bilateral subfoveal neurosensory retinal detachment associated with MEK inhibitor use for metastatic cancer. JAMA Ophthalmol. 2014; 132(8):1005–1009

[26] van Dijk EH, van Herpen CM, Marinkovic M, et al. Serous retinopathy associated with mitogen-activated protein kinase kinase inhibition (binimetinib) for metastatic cutaneous and uveal melanoma. Ophthalmology. 2015; 122(9):1907–1916

[27] Urner-Bloch U, Urner M, Jaberg-Bentele N, Frauchiger AL, Dummer R, Goldinger SM. MEK inhibitor-associated retinopathy (MEKAR) in metastatic melanoma: long-term ophthalmic effects. Eur J Cancer. 2016; 65:130–138

16 Optical Coherence Tomography Angiography and Glaucoma

Gábor Holló

Summary

Vascular dysregulation of the optic nerve head and the peripapillary retina has been proposed for decades as a risk factor for the development and progression of glaucoma, one of the most common reasons of irreversible vision loss and blindness worldwide. Using optical coherence tomography (OCT) angiography, a novel noninvasive functional imaging technology, vessel density and perfusion in various layers of the optic nerve head and the peripapillary retina can be analyzed and measured separately, together with the spatially corresponding en face structural OCT images. OCT angiography allows selective investigation of perfusion in the area of a structural abnormality, which aids accurate diagnosis and may potentially improve our understanding of the pathophysiology of glaucoma and detection of glaucomatous progression. This chapter explains how to understand and evaluate OCT angiography findings of the disc and the peripapillary retina. The reader is introduced to the field, step by step, via clinical cases, starting from findings in healthy eyes and moving on through the characteristics of disc hemorrhages, diffuse and localized glaucomatous disc, and retinal nerve fiber layer damage, to artifacts measurement and the differentiation of glaucomatous and nonglaucomatous perfusion abnormalities.

Keywords: angiovue OCT, optical coherence tomography angiography, disc hemorrhage, en face OCT image, glaucoma, optic nerve head perfusion, retinal nerve fiber layer

16.1 Why Use Optical Coherence Tomography Angiography for Disc Assessment in Glaucoma?

Vascular dysregulation of the optic nerve head and the peripapillary retina is considered as one of the risk factors for the development and progression of open-angle glaucoma.[1] In addition, glaucomatous neuroretinal rim and retinal nerve fiber layer loss is associated with reduced perfusion of the optic nerve head and peripapillary retina in all types of glaucoma. Therefore, in recent decades, various techniques have been used for noninvasive measurement of disc and peripapillary perfusion.[2,3,4] However, vascular structures and their regulation in the disc and the peripapillary retina differ both across the retinal layers and between the retina and choroid, respectively. Noninvasive clinical techniques available in the past decades could not optimally separate perfusion-related information arriving from the different layers.[2,3] This is why research focused on global measures of ocular perfusion, such as retrobulbar perfusion, global retinal oxygenation, and ocular perfusion pressure.[4]

In contrast to the earlier technologies, precise segmentation in modern optical coherence tomography (OCT) makes it possible to accurately separate both the retinal layers (structural information) and the perfusion maps of the individual layers (functional information).[5,6,7,8,9] This enables clinicians to evaluate the corresponding structural and functional information (en face angiograms and en face retinal images), layer by layer, in a noninvasive manner. In practical terms, if a clinician detects an abnormality suggestive for glaucomatous damage, he or she can analyze the layers separately and can focus only on the corresponding structural and functional properties of the layer of interest. The perfusion-related functional data and the structure-related anatomical data provide complementary information.

In addition to qualitative evaluation, precise measurement of perfusion is also important when decreased vascularity or perfusion is investigated in glaucoma. OCT angiography offers options for both qualitative evaluation and quantitative measurement of disc and peripapillary perfusion. The quantitative parameters are vessel density (expressed in % of vessels in the measured area within a well-defined retinal layer) and flow index (the mean decorrelation value of the whole en face angiogram).[5,6,7,8,9] These parameters have been shown to be reproducible both in normal and in glaucomatous eyes; decreased in glaucoma; and their reduction is related to glaucomatous visual field deterioration, retinal nerve fiber layer thickness, inner macular retina thickness, and the stage of glaucoma.[5,6,7,8,9]

It is important to note that advanced glaucomatous disc and retinal nerve fiber layer damage builds up from localized defects; thus, in many early and moderately severe glaucoma cases, only localized neuroretinal rim and retinal nerve fiber layer defects are present. The most typical locations of these localized defects are the inferotemporal and superotemporal disc and peripapillary sectors. When a glaucomatous eye with a localized damage is investigated, it is more informative to measure perfusion in the damaged area separately than to use perfusion data of the whole disc or peripapillary area, because signals arriving from the normal areas diminish the impact of the locally reduced perfusion on the result. In order to offer separate sector analysis for peripapillary vessel density measurement, the AngioVue OCT (Angio-Vue/RTVue-XR Avanti OCT, Optovue Inc., Fremont, CA) employs a recently introduced software version (the Optovue 2015.100.0.33 software version). In this chapter, clinical cases imaged using that instrument and software version are presented. Recently, it has been shown that sector vessel density measured in the retinal nerve fiber layer may decrease prior to the development of clinically significant retinal nerve fiber layer thinning and visual field deterioration, and that it spatially corresponds to the thinned retinal nerve fiber bundles.[8] It is important to emphasize that OCT angiography is based on the detection of moving red blood cells; thus, nonperfused vessels (during strong vasoconstriction), vessels filled with static blood (vessel occlusion), and extravasal blood (bleeding) are not recognized by this technology.

16.2 Determination of Disc and Peripapillary Vessel Density with Optical Coherence Tomography Angiography

The AngioVue OCT obtains amplitude decorrelation angiography images.[5,6,7,8,9] This means that only the moving elements (the circulating red blood cells) provide perfusion-related information. The A-scan rate is 70,000 scans per second, the light source is centered on 840 nm, and a bandwidth of 50 nm is used. Each OCT angiography volume contains 304 × 304 A-scans with two consecutive B-scans captured at each fixed position before proceeding to the next sampling location. Split-spectrum amplitude-decorrelation angiography is used to extract the OCT angiography information. Motion correction to minimize motion artifacts arising from microsaccades and fixation changes is used. OCT angiography information is displayed as the average of the decorrelation values when viewed perpendicularly through the thickness. Six peripapillary sectors (▶ Fig. 16.1) and four en face imaging retinal layers are automatically given by the software. The software-provided peripapillary

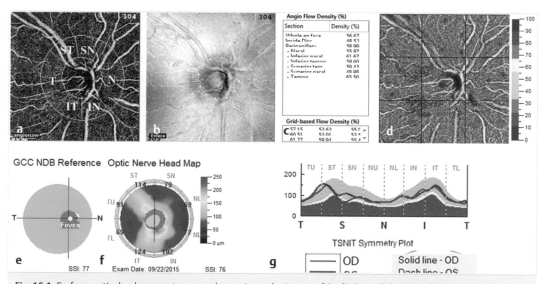

Fig. 16.1 En face optical coherence tomography angiography image of (a,d) the radial peripapillary capillaries layer, (b) en face structural OCT of the retinal nerve fiber layer, (c) the vessel density and flow density measurement report, (e) the ganglion cell complex, (f) the retinal nerve fiber layer map, and (g) the retinal nerve fiber layer thickness symmetry plot of a healthy right eye.

sectors are based on the Garway-Heath map.[10] The corresponding en face vessel density and retinal layers from the vitreous to the choroid are (1) the optic nerve head layer (the innermost layer), (2) the vitreous–retina border, (3) the layer of the radial peripapillary capillaries on the OCT angiography image paired with the retinal nerve fiber layer on the structural retinal image, and (4) the retina–choroid border. Using the "angio structure-function" overview presentation, the subsequent OCT angiography images are shown in the above order in the upper horizontal row, and the corresponding structural images in the lower horizontal row. In OCT angiography for glaucoma assessment, the radial peripapillary capillaries layer is the most important one, since it represents perfusion in the retinal nerve fiber layer. The radial peripapillary capillaries layer is defined as all tissues between the outer limit of the retinal nerve fiber layer and the internal limiting membrane. The other layer that is relevant for the differential diagnosis in glaucoma is the optic nerve head layer spreading from the internal limiting membrane toward the vitreous body in a 150-μm thickness. Usually the $4.5 \times 4.5\ mm^2$ scan size is used for glaucoma investigations. The inner elliptical contour (which defines the optic nerve head) is obtained by automatically fitting an ellipse to the disc margin based on the OCT en face image. The peripapillary area is defined as the area between the inner and outer ellipses. The ring width between the inner and outer elliptical contour lines is usually 0.75 mm. No pupil dilation is needed for optimal image quality (Signal Strength Index > 50).

16.3 Optical Coherence Tomography Angiography of the Healthy Disc

▶ Fig. 16.1 shows disc and peripapillary vessel density measured with OCT angiography in the radial peripapillary capillaries layer, and the corresponding inner macula retinal thickness (ganglion cell complex [GCC]) map, 360-degree retinal nerve fiber layer thickness map, and symmetry graph of the healthy right eye of a 64-year-old female subject. The peripapillary vessel density measurement area (▶ Fig. 16.1a) is subdivided into six sectors: the superotemporal (ST), temporal (T), inferotemporal (IT), inferonasal (IN), nasal (N), and superonasal

(NS) sectors. The corresponding en face structural image (▶ Fig. 16.1b) shows homogeneous normal reflectivity of the retinal nerve fibers in all sectors and in the total image area. Vessel density is 48.5% for the disc area, 59% for the total peripapillary area, and the sector vessel density values range between 55% (nasal) and 65.5% (temporal; ▶ Fig. 16.1c). This range is typical for healthy eyes in the radial peripapillary capillaries layer. Vessels (both the main retinal vessels and the capillary areas) are indicated with yellow and red on the color-coded vessel density map (▶ Fig. 16.1d). The intensity corresponds to the measured signal intensity. In OCT angiography, nonperfusion or poor perfusion is color coded with blue (not present on this image). The GCC map (▶ Fig. 16.1e) and the retinal nerve fiber layer thickness map (▶ Fig. 16.1f) are normal and within normal limits, and the retinal nerve fiber layer thickness symmetry is also within the normal limits (▶ Fig. 16.1g).

16.4 Comparison of Vessel Density between Healthy and End-Stage Glaucomatous Eyes

▶ Fig. 16.2 introduces into OCT angiography findings in glaucoma via the comparison of the vessel density map (▶ Fig. 16.2a), en face structural image (▶ Fig. 16.2b), and color-coded vessel density map (▶ Fig. 16.2c) of the end-stage glaucomatous right eye (cup/disc ratio 1.0) and the corresponding images and maps (▶ Fig. 16.2d, f) of the almost healthy, successfully trabeculectomized ocular hypertensive left eye of the same 48-year-old male patient. On the right eye, diffuse lack of vessels (lack of perfusion) is seen on the density map (▶ Fig. 16.2a). The darkness of the retinal nerve fiber layer (decreased light reflectivity due to diffuse retinal nerve fiber loss; ▶ Fig. 16.2b) is contrasted to the bright retinal nerve fiber layer of the left eye (▶ Fig. 16.2e). The color of the color-coded vessel density map of the right eye is bluish, while it is bright yellow and red for the left eye (▶ Fig. 16.2c,f). The GCC and retinal nerve fiber layer thickness values are outside the normal limits on the right eye and within the normal limits on the left eye (▶ Fig. 16.2g). The peripapillary sector vessel density values range from 40.8 to 47.5% on the right and from 53 to 59% on the left eye in the radial peripapillary capillaries layer.

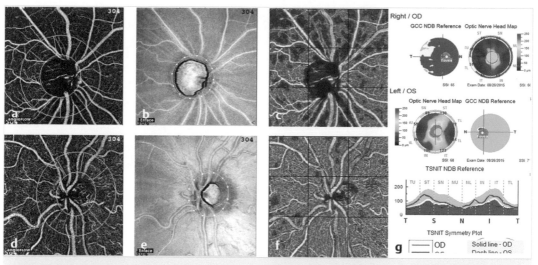

Fig. 16.2 Comparison of vessel density maps obtained with optical coherence tomography angiography in the radial peripapillary capillaries layer of the right eye with **(a–c)** severe diffuse glaucomatous damage and **(d–f)** the almost healthy left eye of the same patient. The ganglion cell complex and retinal nerve fiber layer thickness maps and values are shown **(g)** for both eyes.

16.5 Diffuse Perfusion Damage and Retinal Nerve Fiber Loss in Advanced Glaucoma

▶ Fig. 16.3 and ▶ Fig. 16.4 present disc and peripapillary OCT angiography findings and the corresponding retinal nerve fiber layer, GCC, and visual field alterations in two cases of advanced glaucoma. ▶ Fig. 16.3 shows reduced peripapillary vessel density in the radial peripapillary capillaries layer (right eye; ▶ Fig. 16.3a,c). The most severe loss of perfusion is seen inferotemporally and superotemporally (dark blue nerve fiber bundle type areas on the color-coded vessel density map; ▶ Fig. 16.3c). These particularly severe nerve fiber bundle dropouts (asterisks) are also visible on the en face retinal nerve fiber layer image (▶ Fig. 16.3b) even though the retinal nerve fiber loss (darkness of the retinal nerve fiber layer) is diffuse in the sectors between 12 and 6 o'clock and between 8 and 10 o'clock. It can also be seen that two narrow retinal nerve fiber bundles are somewhat less damaged (arrows): one of them is relatively wide and located inferotemporally at the 7 o'clock position, while the other is narrow and located at the 11 o'clock position (▶ Fig. 16.3b). These relatively intact nerve fiber bundles are represented by relatively well-preserved vessel densities (▶ Fig. 16.3c, arrows). ▶ Fig. 16.3d shows that the inner macula retinal thickness and the retinal nerve fiber layer thickness are outside of the normal limits even in these locations. This shows that the en face perfusion and nerve fiber layer maps allow detection of relatively intact structures embedded in a severely damaged environment, providing options for fine discrimination. The functional consequences are shown on the corresponding visual field (▶ Fig. 16.3e). The visual field shows severe diffuse loss of sensitivity except for an inferior paracentral area spatially corresponding to the intact superotemporal nerve fiber bundle and its unimpaired perfusion, and a larger superior paracentral area spatially corresponding with the wider inferotemporal undamaged nerve fiber bundle and perfusion.

▶ Fig. 16.4 illustrates another case of severe diffuse retinal nerve fiber layer thinning and reduction of perfusion in the radial peripapillary capillaries layer. In this case, a wide papillomacular and a wide inferonasal nerve fiber bundle (▶ Fig. 16.4a) and their vessel densities (▶ Fig. 16.4b,d) are preserved (arrows). The preserved bundles and their unimpaired perfusion are represented by the preserved central and superotemporal visual field areas, respectively (▶ Fig. 16.4c).

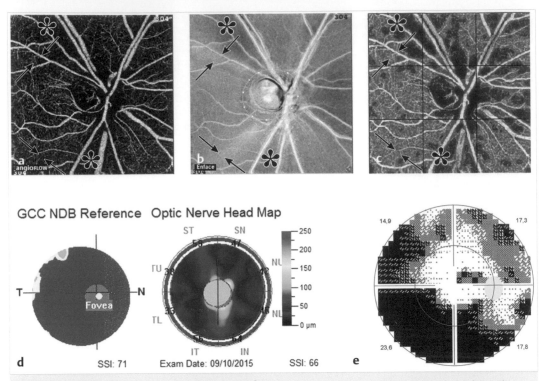

Fig. 16.3 **(a,c)** En face vessel density and **(b)** retinal nerve fiber layer images, **(d)** ganglion cell complex and retinal nerve fiber layer report, and **(e)** the corresponding visual field of an advanced glaucomatous eye with two undamaged narrow nerve fiber bundles (arrows). The most severe retinal nerve fiber bundle dropouts are indicated with asterisks, and the preserved nerve fiber bundles and their positions on the vessel density map are indicated in **(a–c)** with arrows.

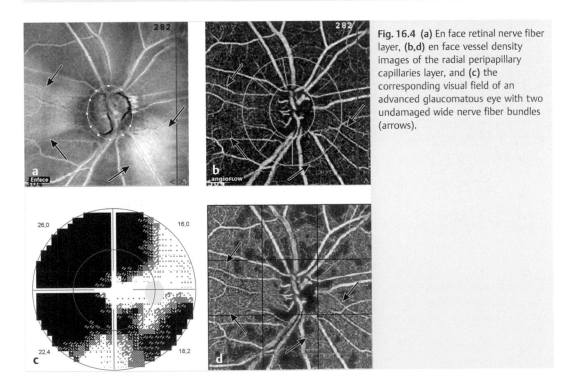

Fig. 16.4 **(a)** En face retinal nerve fiber layer, **(b,d)** en face vessel density images of the radial peripapillary capillaries layer, and **(c)** the corresponding visual field of an advanced glaucomatous eye with two undamaged wide nerve fiber bundles (arrows).

16.6 Localized Perfusion Damage and Retinal Nerve Fiber Loss in Early Glaucoma

▶ Fig. 16.5 shows how useful en face OCT angiography and en face retinal nerve fiber layer imaging can be in relatively early glaucoma (right eye of a 57-year-old female primary open-angle glaucoma patient with Octopus visual field mean defect of 5.2 dB). The visual field shows an extensive superior and a small inferior nasal step (▶ Fig. 16.5a), which spatially correspond to a wide inferotemporal retinal nerve fiber loss and GCC thinning, and a narrow superotemporal nerve fiber layer thinning, respectively (▶ Fig. 16.5b). The en face retinal nerve fiber layer map (▶ Fig. 16.5c) and the color-coded vessel density map (▶ Fig. 16.5d) show the corresponding localized nerve fiber bundle damage and the corresponding perfusion decrease (arrows) embedded in a normal retinal nerve fiber layer and normal retinal perfusion, respectively.

16.7 Discrimination of an Aneurysm from a Deep Disc Hemorrhage in Glaucoma Using Optical Coherence Tomography Angiography

Disc hemorrhages are considered as indicators of ongoing glaucomatous progression. Therefore, intensification of treatment is frequently indicated when disc hemorrhage is detected. However, an aneurysm embedded in the wall of the neuroretinal rim may falsely suggest a deep hemorrhage.[11] Distinguishing between an aneurism and a deep disc hemorrhage may be particularly difficult when the eye does in fact suffer from glaucoma, and the patient is seen for the first time by the ophthalmologist. ▶ Fig. 16.6 illustrates the usefulness of OCT angiography for the differentiation between an aneurysm and a true disc hemorrhage in glaucoma. The vessel density maps (▶ Fig. 16.6a,c) show the

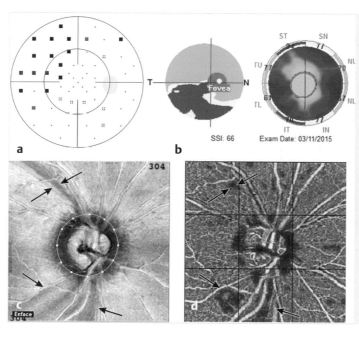

Fig. 16.5 (a) Visual field, **(b)** ganglion cell complex and retinal nerve fiber layer thickness report, **(c)** the corresponding en face retinal nerve fiber layer and **(d)** vessel density maps of a relatively early glaucoma eye. The damaged retinal nerve fiber bundles are indicated with arrows.

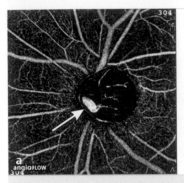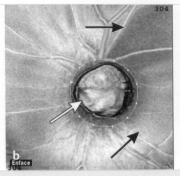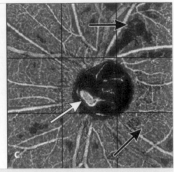

Fig. 16.6 **(a,c)** Vessel density maps and **(b)** en face retinal nerve fiber layer images of a glaucoma eye with a vascular aneurysm resembling a deep disc hemorrhage (white arrows). The most severe retinal nerve fiber layer damage is indicated with black arrows.

high flow in the aneurysm located inferonasally (white arrow). The aneurysm cannot be recognized as such on the en face nerve fiber layer map (► Fig. 16.6b); therefore, its red color may suggest bleeding during ophthalmoscopy. The true nerve fiber layer thinning and perfusion damage are predominantly superotemporal and temporal (► Fig. 16.6b,c, black arrows). As indicated earlier in this chapter, true hemorrhages are not detected by OCT angiography owing to the lack of movement of the red blood cells.[11] In contrast, aneurysms are characterized by high blood flow and high signal intensity, which facilitate easy discrimination of the two entities.

16.8 Optical Coherence Tomography Angiography Signs of a True Disc Hemorrhage

► Fig. 16.7 and ► Fig. 16.8 show the OCT angiography characteristics of disc hemorrhages[11] in advanced and early glaucoma, respectively. In ► Fig. 16.7, the disc hemorrhage is located at the 9 o'clock position in the left eye (white arrows). While it is detectable on all en face structural maps (► Fig. 16.7a), only a minimal shadow effect (reduced signal intensity) is seen on the corresponding vessel density maps (► Fig. 16.7a). The bleeding is located next to a severe and wide nerve fiber bundle thinning, indicating that the progression of this localized damage is ongoing. The corresponding visual field (► Fig. 16.7b), en face retinal nerve fiber layer map (► Fig. 16.7c), and color-coded vessel density map (► Fig. 16.7d) show severe glaucomatous damage.

► Fig. 16.8 shows a disc hemorrhage at the 7 o'clock position in early glaucoma (right eye). The hemorrhage (white arrow) is located next to a narrow nerve fiber bundle defect (black arrows), suggesting its ongoing progression. The hemorrhage is easier to detect on the innermost layer en face structural image (in the optic nerve head layer) but remains undetectable on the vessel density maps, in which decreased perfusion spatially corresponding to the nerve fiber bundle dropout is clearly visible (► Fig. 16.8a). The corresponding GCC and retinal nerve fiber layer thinning (► Fig. 16.8b), vessel density map (► Fig. 16.8c), en face retinal nerve fiber layer map (► Fig. 16.8d), and color-coded vessel density map (► Fig. 16.8e) show deterioration corresponding to the nerve fiber bundle defect.

16.9 Detection of Artifacts Resembling Perfusion Damage and Nerve Fiber Loss

Vitreous floaters may cause shadow effects when retinal nerve fiber layer and inner macula retinal thickness are measured. A similar effect is also not uncommon in OCT angiography. Without a detailed clinical examination, the decreased signal intensity due to unrecognized vitreous floaters may cause a diagnostic error. The influence of vitreous floaters is particularly problematic when their shape is similar to that of a nerve fiber bundle. ► Fig. 16.9 shows the effect of a superotemporally located vitreous floater shaped like a nerve fiber bundle in a glaucomatous right eye, its influence on the OCT angiography result, and how this

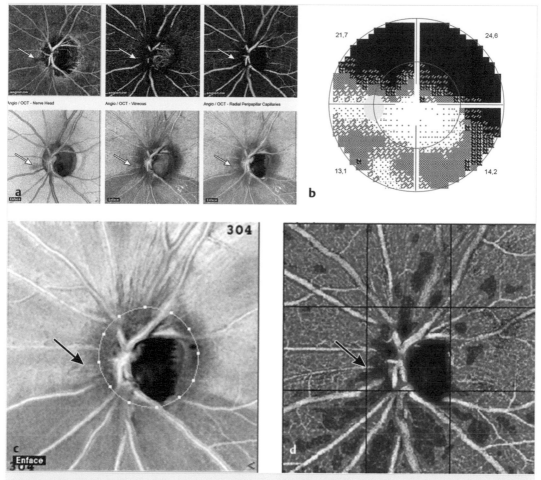

Fig. 16.7 Superficial disc hemorrhage (arrow) in advanced glaucoma. **(a)** Overview of the en face optical coherence tomography angiography and retina layers, **(b)** visual field, **(c)** retinal nerve fiber layer, and **(d)** vessel density map of the radial peripapillary capillaries layer.

artifact can be distinguished from true damage. ▶ Fig. 16.9a shows how similar this shadow artifact (white arrow) is to a true nerve fiber bundle type perfusion loss, for all en face vessel density layers. The nature of this artifact is somewhat easier to recognize on the corresponding en face structural images. The vessel density measurement maps (▶ Fig. 16.9b,d) and the en face retinal nerve fiber layer map (▶ Fig. 16.9c) all suggest a severe nerve fiber bundle type defect superotemporally (artifact) and inferotemporally (true damage). When the patient is reexamined later (after the floater has moved away from the image area), the shadow effect is no longer visible, while the true nerve fiber bundle damage (black arrows)

and the spatially corresponding decrease of vessel density remain unchanged (▶ Fig. 16.9e).

16.10 Differential Diagnosis of Glaucoma Using Optical Coherence Tomography Angiography

A detailed clinical investigation of the eye and patient is essential before OCT angiography findings are used for making a clinical diagnosis or reaching a decision on disease stability. OCT angiography findings are not disease specific; thus, distinguishing

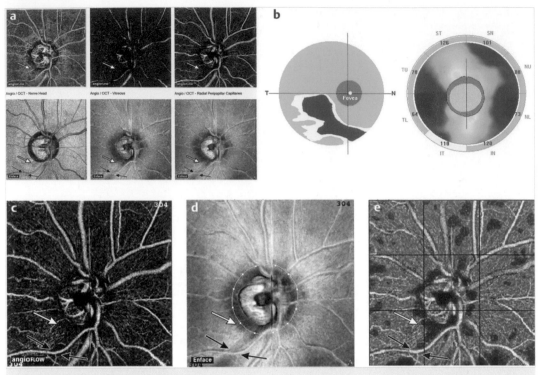

Fig. 16.8 **(a,c–e)**Superficial disc hemorrhage in early glaucoma (white arrow), the position of the neighboring nerve fiber bundle defect (black arrows), and **(b)** the corresponding ganglion cell complex and retinal nerve fiber layer maps.

vessel density decrease due to glaucoma from decrease caused by other diseases is not possible without clinical evaluation. ▶ Fig. 16.10 shows en face vessel density and en face retinal images (▶ Fig. 16.10a) of a right eye suffering from severe optic nerve head pallor due to an earlier optic neuritis. The lack of disc and peripapillary perfusion on the color-coded vessel density map (▶ Fig. 16.10c) is very similar to that seen in end-stage glaucoma (▶ Fig. 16.2, right eye). The visual field damage is also severe and has a nerve fiber bundle shape (▶ Fig. 16.10b). ▶ Fig. 16.11 shows a case of acute nonarteritic anterior ischemic optic neuropathy (right eye). The lack of perfusion around the inferior and nasal border of the disc on all en face perfusion maps (white arrows) spatially correspond to the edema seen in the same sectors on all en face structural images (▶ Fig. 16.11a, black arrows) and the edema visible on the disc photograph (▶ Fig. 16.11b, arrows). The visual field shows corresponding superior damage (▶ Fig. 16.11c), and the measured retinal nerve fiber layer thickness is abnormally elevated inferiorly and nasally compared to that of the healthy fellow eye (▶ Fig. 16.11d).

Compression by optic disc drusen (arrows) may also cause reduced peripapillary perfusion and nerve fiber loss (▶ Fig. 16.12, arrows, right eye of a 39-year-old male patient). ▶ Fig. 16.12a shows the significant inferior GCC and retinal nerve fiber layer thinning between the 12 and 7 o'clock positions. The spatially corresponding retinal nerve fiber loss and decreased vessel density are shown in ▶ Fig. 16.12b and c, respectively.

Myelinated retinal nerve fibers may also resemble decreased perfusion in the radial peripapillary capillaries layer within the area of the myelinated fibers.[12] This is due to the volume of the myelin sheaths, which can dislocate the fibers toward the vitreous body. At the same time, this change of position may result in increased OCT angiography vessel density in the optic nerve head layer within the myelinated area.[12] ▶ Fig. 16.13 shows a different OCT angiography presentation of the effect of myelinated nerve fibers, and the appearance of the Zinn–Haller vascular ring, on the same eye. The myelinated fibers are located superiorly (▶ Fig. 16.13a, black arrows). They cause decreased vessel density on all en face OCT angiography

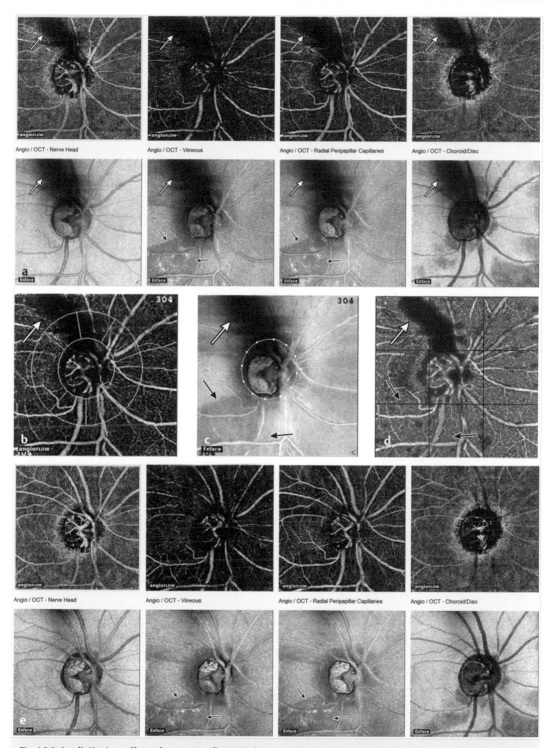

Fig. 16.9 (a–d) Shadow effect of a vitreous floater (white arrow) imitating a retinal nerve fiber bundle defect in a glaucomatous eye, and (e) the same area after the vitreous floater moved away from the original position. The true retinal nerve fiber layer damage area is indicated with black arrows in **(a,c–e)**.

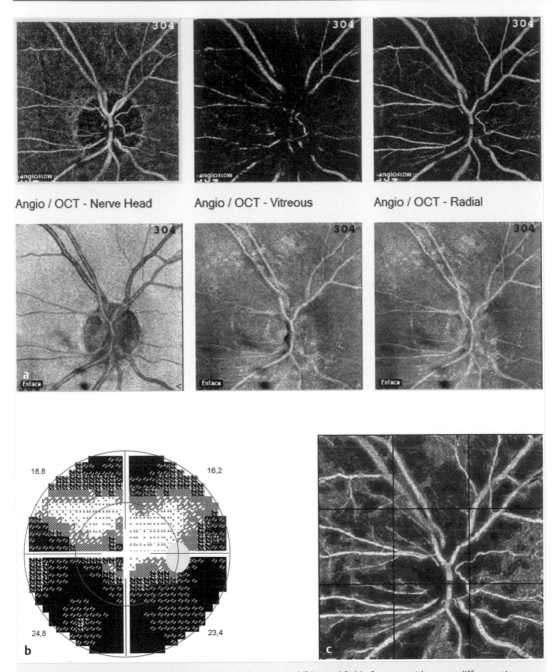

Fig. 16.10 (a,c) En face OCT angiography and retinal maps, and (b) visual field of an eye with severe diffuse optic nerve head pallor. The detailed explanation is given in the text.

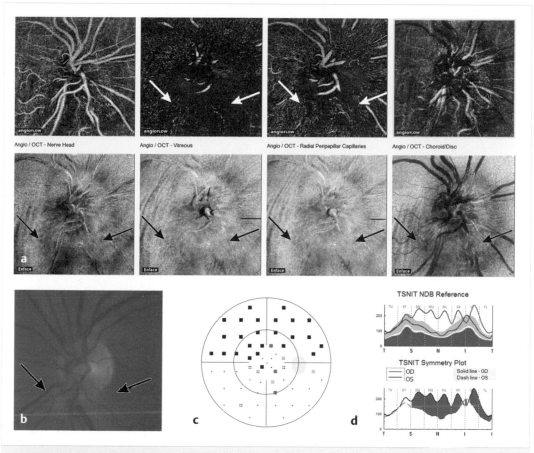

Fig. 16.11 **(a)** En face OCT angiography and retinal images, **(b)** disc photography, **(c)** visual field, and **(d)** retinal nerve fiber layer thickness symmetry plot of an eye with acute nonarteritic anterior ischemic optic neuropathy. The area of nonperfusion is indicated with white arrows in **(a)**, and the area of disc swelling with black arrows in **(a,b)**.

layers, and appear as an additional volume on the en face structural images (▶ Fig. 16.13b). In the optic nerve head layer (▶ Fig. 16.13c), the deep peripapillary arterial ring (the Zinn–Haller ring) is clearly visible on the vessel density map (white arrows). This ring is incomplete and less visible in most eyes. The myelinated nerve fibers are also visible on the corresponding enlarged en face structural map (▶ Fig. 16.13d). The vessel density is reduced due to the myelin sheaths in the area of the myelinated fibers (▶ Fig. 16.13e). In the radial peripapillary capillaries layer, the disc and peripapillary vessel density is reduced within the area of the myelinated fibers (▶ Fig. 16.13f–h), but the distribution of the decreased vessel density is different compared to that observed in the more superficial layer (▶ Fig. 16.13e). These findings and the previously published case report[12] suggest that OCT angiography results need to be interpreted with caution when myelinated retinal nerve fibers are present.

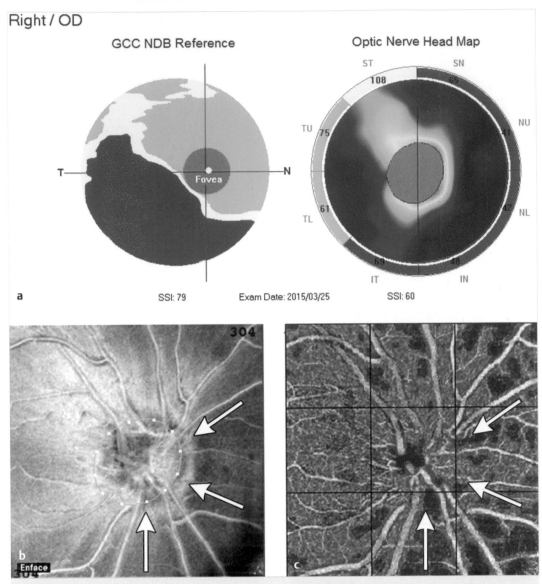

Fig. 16.12 **(a)** Ganglion cell complex and retinal nerve fiber layer thickness map, **(b)** en face retinal nerve fiber layer, and **(c)** vessel density map of the radial peripapillary capillaries layer of an eye with extensive retinal nerve fiber loss due to optic nerve head drusen (arrows).

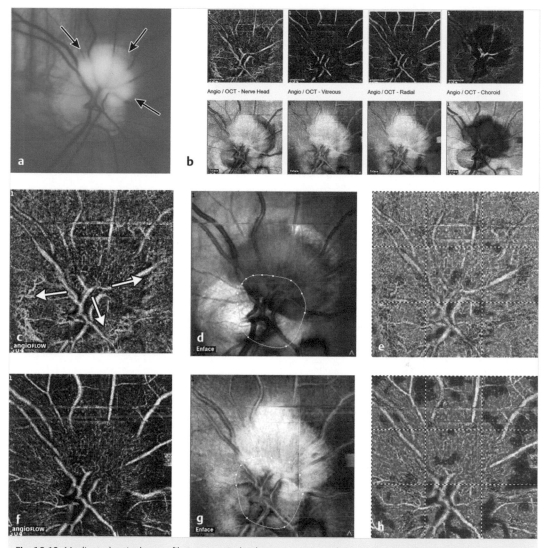

Fig. 16.13 Myelinated retinal nerve fibers on optical coherence tomography angiography. **(a)** Myelinated retinal nerve fibers with optic nerve photography (black arrows), **(b)** en face optical coherence tomography angiography and retinal layers, **(c,e)** vessel density, **(d)** retinal image of the optic nerve head layer, **(f,h)** vessel density, and **(g)** en face image of the radial peripapillary capillaries layer. The Zinn–Haller vascular ring is indicated with white arrows in **(c)**.

16.11 The Future of Optical Coherence Tomography Angiography in Glaucoma Research and Clinics

Clinical use of OCT angiography in glaucoma started only 1 year ago. It has already been shown that peripapillary vessel density may decrease before retinal nerve fiber layer thickness deviates significantly from the normal range. This suggests that OCT angiography may gain importance in early diagnosis of glaucoma. Currently, no information is available on the usefulness of OCT angiography in early detection of glaucomatous progression. This is due to the short time that has elapsed since the introduction of the method in clinical practice. Peripapillary sector vessel density values seem to be particularly informative for the quantitative characterization of glaucomatous perfusion loss. Therefore, refinement of the sector borders, or an option for custom-made definitions of sector borders offered by the manufacturer, may increase the accuracy of the method. It is unquestionable that OCT angiography in glaucoma will develop rapidly in the upcoming years.

16.12 Disclosure

Gábor Holló is an unpaid consultant of Optovue, Inc.

References

[1] Quaranta L, Katsanos A, Russo A, Riva I. 24-hour intraocular pressure and ocular perfusion pressure in glaucoma. Surv Ophthalmol. 2013; 58(1):26–41

[2] Holló G, van den Berg TJ, Greve EL. Scanning laser Doppler flowmetry in glaucoma. Int Ophthalmol. 1996–1997; 20(1–3): 63–70

[3] Holló G, Greve EL, van den Berg TJ, Vargha P. Evaluation of the peripapillary circulation in healthy and glaucoma eyes with scanning laser Doppler flowmetry. Int Ophthalmol. 1996–1997; 20(1–3):71–77

[4] Pinto AL, Willekens K, Van Keer K, et al. Ocular blood flow in glaucoma: the Leuven Eye Study. Acta Ophthalmol. 2016; 94 (6):592–8

[5] Liu L, Jia Y, Takusagawa HL, et al. Optical coherence tomography angiography of the peripapillary retina in glaucoma. JAMA Ophthalmol. 2015; 133(9):1045–1052

[6] Wang X, Jiang C, Ko T, et al. Correlation between optic disc perfusion and glaucomatous severity in patients with open-angle glaucoma: an optical coherence tomography angiography study. Graefes Arch Clin Exp Ophthalmol. 2015; 253(9):1557–1564

[7] Pechauer AD, Jia Y, Liu L, Gao SS, Jiang C, Huang D. Optical coherence tomography angiography of peripapillary retinal blood flow response to hyperoxia. Invest Ophthalmol Vis Sci. 2015; 56(5):3287–3291

[8] Holló G. Vessel density calculated from OCT angiography in 3 peripapillary sectors in normal, ocular hypertensive, and glaucoma eyes. Eur J Ophthalmol. 2016; 26(3):e42–e45

[9] Lévêque P-M, Zéboulon P, Brasnu E, Baudouin C, Labbé A. Optic disc vascularization in glaucoma: value of spectral-domain optical coherence tomography angiography. J Ophthalmol. 2016; 2016:6956717

[10] Garway-Heath DF, Poinoosawmy D, Fitzke FW, Hitchings RA. Mapping the visual field to the optic disc in normal tension glaucoma eyes. Ophthalmology. 2000; 107(10):1809–1815

[11] Holló G. Combined use of Doppler OCT and en face OCT functions for discrimination of an aneurysm in the lamina cribrosa from a disc hemorrhage. Eur J Ophthalmol. 2015; 26 (1):e8–e10

[12] Holló G. Influence of myelinated retinal nerve fibers on retinal vessel density measurement with AngioVue OCT angiography. Int Ophthalmol. 2016; 36(6):915–919

17 Optical Coherence Tomography Angiography and Anterior Segment Vasculature

Christophe Baudouin, Stephanie Hayek, and Adil El Maftouhi

Summary

Optical coherence tomography angiography (OCTA) is actually a revolution for retinal diseases and now shows similar potential for anterior segment vasculature. Indeed, the ocular surface and iris vasculature are not easily accessible, and fluorescein angiography is rarely performed for such evaluations and cannot be easily repeated. OCTA is a totally noninvasive technique; it can be repeated over time as often as needed and may thus offer an incredible potential for following disease evolution and monitoring treatment efficacy. Corneal neovascularization is a potentially severe complication in various corneal diseases and a high-risk factor for corneal rejection following keratoplasty. The conjunctiva assessment, the tumor development, and bleb formation after glaucoma surgery are examples of the numerous potentialities of OCTA. Early detection of iris neovascularization is also a major goal when monitoring ischemic diseases of the retina, and is now easily accessible with OCTA. Additionally, as OCTA relies on moving structures and not optical densities, the clear discrepancy between slit-lamp examination and vascular density in OCTA strongly suggests that this new tool not only targets blood vessels, but also a totally nonvisible parallel vascular network, namely lymphatic vessels. A new semiology of the anterior segment is probably in our hands and will certainly benefit from future sustained and continuous technical progress.

Keywords: optical coherence tomography angiography, anterior segment, vasculature, cornea, conjunctiva, iris, rubeosis iridis, lymphatics, glaucoma surgery

17.1 Introduction

Currently, the assessment of the anterior segment vasculature is constrained to slit-lamp photography or invasive techniques using fluorescein or indocyanine green (ICG) angiography.[1,2] Optical coherence tomography angiography (OCTA) has been initially applied to evaluate posterior segment vascular conditions such as retinopathies or choroidal neovascularization.[3] In this chapter, we try to demonstrate OCTA as a new valuable technique for the anterior segment of the eye. We evaluated this new imaging technique in describing abnormal corneal neovascularization in patients with various corneal disease.[4,5,6] In conjunctival and corneal diseases, invasion of the cornea by vessels is often the hint or initiator of more serious diseases. Therefore, the study of vessels is important to understand disease process and to follow the treatment response. Moreover, OCTA has opened a new field of investigation in pathologies where vasculature is only accessible through invasive techniques with potential risks for the patients. This is a new semiology that is now arising and will benefit from further technical improvements.

17.2 Principles of Optical Coherence Tomography Angiography for the Front of the Eye

We used the commercially available spectral-domain OCT RT XR Avanti with the AngioVue software (Optovue, Inc., Fremont, CA). The instrument used for OCTA images was based on the AngioVue Imaging System to obtain amplitude-decorrelation angiography images. The Avanti OCT operates at an 840-nm wavelength range and generates 70,000 axial-scans per second. Each OCTA volume contains 304 × 304 A-scans with two consecutive B-scans captured at each fixed position before proceeding to the next sampling location. Split-spectrum amplitude-decorrelation angiography (SSADA) was used to extract the OCTA information.[7] To obtain a scan of the anterior segment, we used the AngioVue OCTA system using the anterior segment optical adaptor lens (L-CAM). A specific anterior module (angiocornea) was used to perform anterior segment scans. The best scans were processed automatically to reduce motion artifacts such as transversal saccadic and residual axial motion in the internal software. Using the CAM lens, the scan size was 6 × 6 mm and was obtained with rapid acquisition (4–5 seconds per scan).

17.3 Technical Issues

Despite continuous improvements, the quality of the anterior segment scans is still not as good as the retinal images even after reducing motion artifacts. Anterior segment OCTA does not tolerate any eye movement of the patient because even micromovements create transverse artifacts on the final images. Therefore, scans cannot be performed when patients are unable to fixate, or have continuous eye or eyelid movements such as nystagmus or symptoms causing abnormal blinking rate or blepharospasm. Another issue of the anterior segment module is that it still does not allow quantitative analyses. In particular, it does not provide numerical data about corneal or conjunctival flow areas as it may allow at the level of the posterior segment.

17.4 Optical Coherence Tomography Angiography in Corneal Diseases

Scans were performed for various corneal diseases, such as corneal neovascularization in corneal graft rejection, pterygium, postherpetic, fungal keratitis, or limbal stem cell deficiency. Evaluation of abnormal corneal and limbal vessels is important considering the visual impairment it may cause. One major interest is to use the anterior segment module of the OCTA to evaluate corneal neovascularization, as new blood vessels may accompany or even precede graft rejection, and are strongly associated with immune and inflammatory reactions. Subtle changes may be missed or underestimated by slit-lamp examination, which makes OCTA a major tool for early evaluation of such threatening complication. As seen in ▸ Fig. 17.1 and ▸ Fig. 17.2, OCTA is able to clearly define the corneal vessels invading the corneal graft, in a much more visible way than on the slit-lamp photographs. It also shows clearly the abnormal vascular loops and the demarcation between normal and abnormal vessels. OCTA shows the vessel organization at the graft interface; in particular, it precisely shows the vessels passing the graft–host junction (▸ Fig. 17.1d).

OCTA can also be extremely useful to describe abnormal neovascularization in stromal keratitis, especially when stromal scarring causes loss of transparency and masks new blood vessels. ▸ Fig. 17.3 shows a central corneal lesion secondary to herpes

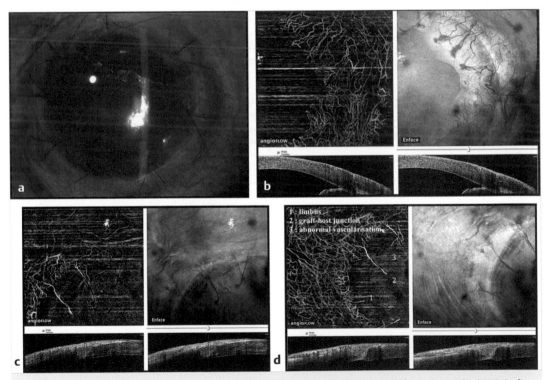

Fig. 17.1 (a) Slit-lamp image of corneal graft rejection. (b) Optical coherence tomography angiography (OCTA) of corneal graft rejection in the nasal quadrant, (c) superior quadrant, (d) temporal quadrant.

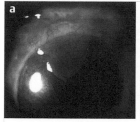
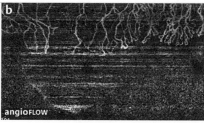

Fig. 17.2 (a) Slit-lamp image of corneal graft rejection with abnormal corneal vessels on the superior quadrant. (b) Optical coherence tomography angiography clearly showing superior conjunctival vessels invading the corneal graft: abnormal vascular loops typical of active neovascularization.

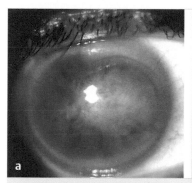
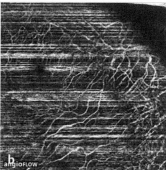
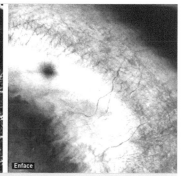

Fig. 17.3 (a) Slit-lamp image of postherpetic stromal keratitis. Note the low density of visible vessels. (b) Optical coherence tomography angiography (OCTA) showing the abnormal vessels invading the corneal stroma. Note the discrepancy between slit-lamp or infrared images and vessel density in OCTA.

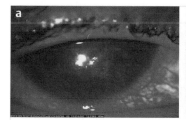
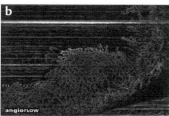

Fig. 17.4 (a) Slit-lamp image of infectious keratitis with intense neovascularization. (b) Optical coherence tomography angiography showing blood vessels invading the cornea. Note the extremely high density of tightly and homogeneously arranged vessels.

simplex virus in a 45-year-old man with a long history of recurrent stromal keratitis in his right eye. The slit-lamp photography shows epithelial and stromal edema, whereas OCTA images show more precisely the abnormal vessels. ▶ Fig. 17.4 shows clearly on the OCTA scan a penetrating vessel in the stroma secondary to a fungal ulcer, 1 month after treatment. These findings are of particular importance when persistence of infection is suspected in inflammatory eyes in which keratoplasty is envisaged.

17.5 OCTA for Conjunctival Vessel Assessment: Application in Glaucoma Surgery

OCTA is also helpful for documenting the vascular patterns in conjunctival inflammation or wound healing, especially after glaucoma surgery when monitoring bleb formation and evaluating proper functioning of the filtering bleb. To obtain an image of the conjunctiva with OCTA, the subject has to look toward the opposite side of the scan. For example, the subject has to look toward the nasal side if the temporal side of the conjunctiva is scanned. A custom software algorithm is used to identify conjunctival boundaries and generate depth-resolved en face angiograms by maximal flow projection. The OCT angiograms revealed rich vascular density in the conjunctiva (▶ Fig. 17.5).

As previously shown with fluorescein angiography description of blebs,[8] OCTA can also be useful to describe conjunctival vessels after glaucoma surgery. It may have a potential as an investigative tool to study the conjunctival and episcleral vasculature changes after trabeculectomy or deep

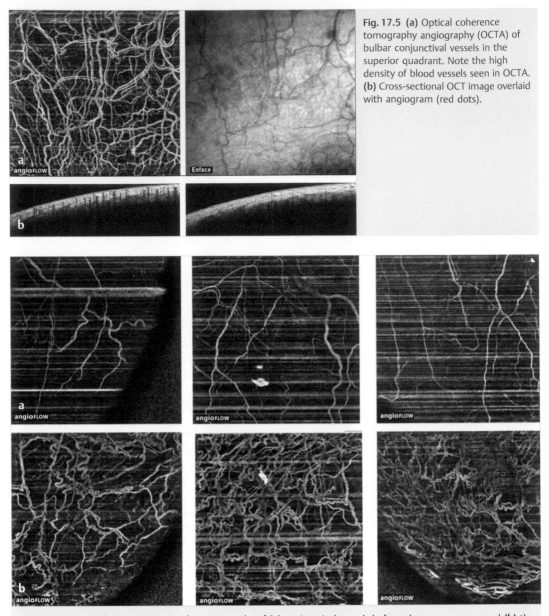

Fig. 17.5 **(a)** Optical coherence tomography angiography (OCTA) of bulbar conjunctival vessels in the superior quadrant. Note the high density of blood vessels seen in OCTA. **(b)** Cross-sectional OCT image overlaid with angiogram (red dots).

Fig. 17.6 Optical coherence tomography angiography of **(a)** conjunctival vessels before glaucoma surgery and **(b)** the bleb vessels at 7 days postoperative.

sclerectomy, with the major advantages of being totally noninvasive and repeated as frequently as desired. ► Fig. 17.6 clearly shows the conjunctival and subconjunctival vasculature before surgery, and the vessel development and reorganization within and around the bleb at 1 week postoperative: the vasculature alterations include much higher vascular density, dilated and tortuous vessels, and vascular anastomoses. When correlating slit-lamp images to OCTA, as in ► Fig. 17.7, the vasculature seen on the OCTA images is much denser and clearly visible. It may correspond to profound scleral vessels that are not visible on slit lamp or it could be hypothesized as being different structures from blood vessels, namely, lymphatics. Conversely, in post-mitomycin C ischemic blebs (► Fig. 17.8), OCTA shows avascular zones. Avascular spaces between dense vascular networks may

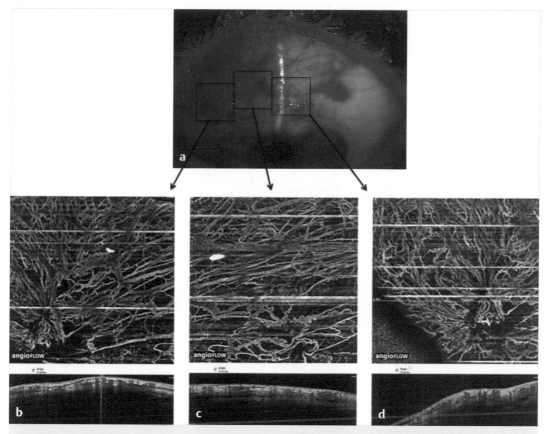

Fig. 17.7 optical coherence tomography angiography of conjunctival vessels at the bleb level, 1 month postoperative. **(a)** Slit-lamp photograph of the bleb. **(b)** Temporal section of the bleb. **(c)** Center of the bleb. **(d)** Nasal section of the bleb.

reflect the presence of aqueous humor and are therefore indicating proper wound healing and bleb formation. Absence of free vessel intervals and increased vessel density may reflect inflammatory states and early stages of bleb scarring and loss of functionality (▶ Fig. 17.9).

17.6 Iris Vessels

The microvasculature of the iris has been previously studied by fluorescein angiography,[9] a technique that is minimally invasive but may expose the patient to potentially severe allergic reactions and cannot be easily repeated. OCTA of the iris appears to be able to demonstrate vessels difficult to photograph or to clinically observe by slit-lamp examination. To obtain such images of the iris, the patient has to look straight ahead while OCTA images are acquired. The iris angiograms show radial iris vessel patterns in normal light-colored

eyes (▶ Fig. 17.10). In darker iris, the pigment produces shadowing and artifacts that obscure the vasculature. The major interest of iris angiograms is to evaluate rubeosis iridis (▶ Fig. 17.11 and ▶ Fig. 17.12). Early stages can be observed much more easily than with the slit lamp, and repeated measures can be performed. This may be of major interest after retinal vein occlusion or in diabetic retinopathy, which iris new blood vessels witness severe ischemic retinopathies, leading to extremely threatening complications, such as neovascular glaucoma.

17.7 Blood or Lymphatic Vessels?

Corneal and conjunctival lymphangiogenesis play a critical role in malignant, inflammatory, or infectious disorders of the ocular surface, and in corneal

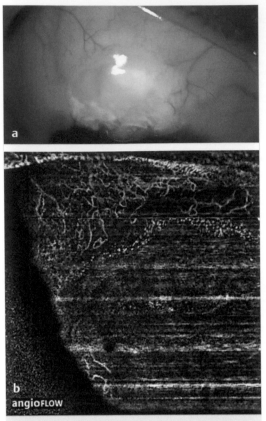

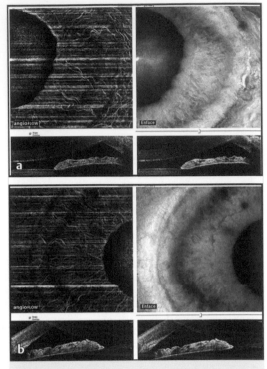

Fig. 17.10 (a,b) En face iris vasculature optical coherence tomography angiography (OCTA) showing normal iris vessels (left). Bottom: The iris vessels (red dots) are overlaid on the cross-sectional OCT image.

Fig. 17.8 (a) Correlated slit-lamp photography and **(b)** optical coherence tomography angiography image of conjunctival vessels in a mitomycin C bleb, showing no vessels in the cystic area.

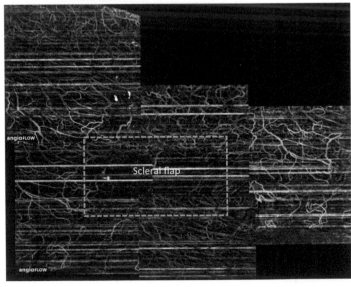

Fig. 17.9 Reconstruction of a filtering bleb with optical coherence tomography angiography 6 × 6 mm scans to recreate the entire bleb.

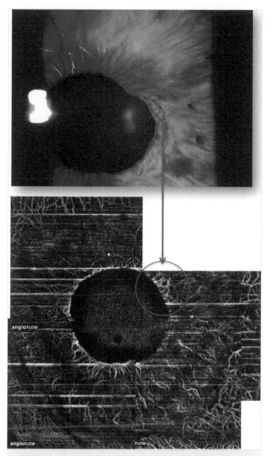

Fig. 17.11 Optical coherence tomography angiography showing rubeosis iridis correlated to slit-lamp photography.

graft rejection. There is no recognized method to visualize and analyze the lymphatic vessels of the human cornea and conjunctiva in vivo. But the recent use of ICG to image lymphatic vessels in the cornea[10] and conjunctiva[11] raises the possibility of applying OCTA to detect lymphatics. As seen on many figures of anterior segment OCTA combined with slit-lamp photography, it is remarkable that the vascular density is much more significant on OCTA scans than on slit lamp. This suggests that the vessels not visible on slit lamp may correspond to a vascular network of different nature, such as lymphatics. Indeed, the principle of OCTA relies on reconstruction of moving elements, and not color or optical density. Therefore, it is quite possible that OCTA provides in a totally noninvasive way images of a nonvisible vascular network consisting of lymphatics.

17.8 Conclusion

This new imaging technique of the anterior segment may be highly useful for an objective evaluation of corneal, conjunctival, or iris vasculature or neovascularization. Although fluorescein and ICG angiography are useful in describing anterior segment vasculature, these potentially invasive techniques are not performed in routine for the anterior segment evaluation, and can hardly be repeated over time to assess disease evolution or treatment response. Therefore, OCTA offers a new clinical tool in a large variety of anterior segment diseases with multiple potential applications, which are expected to increase with further technical improvements, like the ones already available for assessing the retinal vasculature.

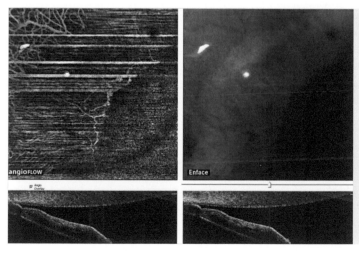

Fig. 17.12 Iris optical coherence tomography angiography showing rubeosis iridis.

References

[1] Kirwan RP, Zheng Y, Tey A, Anijeet D, Sueke H, Kaye SB. Quantifying changes in corneal neovascularization using fluorescein and indocyanine green angiography. Am J Ophthalmol. 2012; 154(5):850–858.e2

[2] Easty DL, Bron AJ. Fluorescein angiography of the anterior segment. Its value in corneal disease. Br J Ophthalmol. 1971; 55(10):671–682

[3] Chalam KV, Sambhav K. Optical coherence tomography angiography in retinal diseases. J Ophthalmic Vis Res. 2016; 11(1):84–92

[4] Ang M, Cai Y, MacPhee B, et al. Optical coherence tomography angiography and indocyanine green angiography for corneal vascularisation. Br J Ophthalmol. 2016, Nov; 100(11):1557–1563

[5] Ang M, Cai Y, Shahipasand S, et al. En face optical coherence tomography angiography for corneal neovascularisation. Br J Ophthalmol. 2016; 100(5):616–621

[6] Ang M, Sim DA, Keane PA, et al. Optical coherence tomography angiography for anterior segment vasculature imaging. Ophthalmology. 2015; 122(9):1740–1747

[7] Huang D, Jia Y, Gao SS, Lumbroso B, Rispoli M. Optical coherence tomography angiography using the Optovue device. Dev Ophthalmol. 2016; 56:6–12

[8] Alsagoff Z, Chew PT, Chee CK, Wong JS, Aung T. Indocyanine green anterior segment angiography for studying conjunctival vascular changes after trabeculectomy. Clin Experiment Ophthalmol. 2001; 29(1):22–26

[9] Parodi MB, Bondel E, Russo D, Ravalico G. Iris indocyanine green videoangiography in diabetic iridopathy. Br J Ophthalmol. 1996; 80(5):416–419

[10] Romano V, Steger B, Zheng Y, Ahmad S, Willoughby CE, Kaye SB. Angiographic and in vivo confocal microscopic characterization of human corneal blood and presumed lymphatic neovascularization: a pilot study. Cornea. 2015; 34 (11):1459–1465

[11] Freitas-Neto CA, Costa RA, Kombo N, et al. Subconjunctival indocyanine green identifies lymphatic vessels. JAMA Ophthalmol. 2015; 133(1):102–104

18 The Future of Optical Coherence Tomography Angiography

Emily D. Cole, Eric M. Moult, Eduardo A. Novais, James G. Fujimoto, and Nadia K. Waheed

Summary

There are exciting advances being made in the applications of optical coherence tomography angiography (OCTA) to the diagnosis and monitoring of ophthalmic disease, ranging from the development of new swept-source OCT devices to the automated, quantitative analysis of OCTA images using novel algorithms. Doppler OCT also represents a promising method to noninvasively quantify blood flow to the optic nerve. Improvement in the hardware and software components of OCTA, as well as a standardized interpretation of these images and their artifacts by ophthalmologists, is important for the further development of this imaging modality.

Keywords: swept-source optical coherence tomography angiography, doppler optical coherence tomography, quantitative optical coherence tomography angiography

18.1 Spectral Domain and Swept-Source Optical Coherence Tomography

Optical coherence tomography angiography (OCTA), with the ability to visualize vasculature in vivo without the injection of dye, represents an exciting advancement in the field of ophthalmic imaging. Over the next few years, there are likely to be rapid advances in both the software and the hardware components of this technology, which will enhance our ability to visualize ophthalmic structures in health and disease. In this chapter, we will touch upon some of the advancements that are on the horizon for OCTA technology.

Spectral-domain optical coherence tomography (SD-OCT) devices are widely used to evaluate retinal and choroidal diseases and form the majority of the machines that are available to clinicians for performing OCTA. Currently, all the commercially available OCTA devices are spectral-domain devices, with the exception of the Topcon DRI Triton, which is a swept-source optical coherence tomography (SS-OCT) device. However, visualization of vascular structures beneath the retinal pigment epithelium (RPE) using shorter wavelength spectral-domain devices may be limited, which will be discussed later in this chapter. Longer wavelength SS-OCT technology may provide a solution for imaging through media opacities and better visualizing the choroid.[1,2,3,4]

Like SD-OCT, SS-OCT is a variation of Fourier-domain OCT.[5,6,7,8] The hardware of SS-OCT differs from SD-OCT in several ways, including the light source, bulk optics components, and photodetection devices. Current ophthalmic SS-OCT light sources use a wavelength centered at approximately 1 µm that sweeps across a band of wavelengths. SS-OCT utilizes a point photodetector, while SD-OCT uses a spectrometer consisting of a diffraction grating and a detector array or a line-scan camera.[9] Both SD-OCT and SS-OCT devices have been used in OCTA configurations to visualize vasculature in vivo.[7,8] New commercially available SS-OCTA devices are likely better able to visualize the choroid and choriocapillaris. However, this is not only due to the swept-source nature of the devices.[10,11] The wavelength of the light source also plays an important role in the visualization of vasculature on OCTA, particularly at deeper locations beneath the RPE. Longer-wavelength light sources currently in use in swept-source devices are capable of improved visualization of the choriocapillaris and choroid and improved immunity to ocular opacity. Thus, they may be useful for improved visualization of choroidal neovascularization (CNV), especially the sub-RPE components of the membrane. One trade-off of longer wavelengths, however, is that longer wavelengths have lower axial resolution compared to shorter wavelengths. In a comparative study, a prototype long-wavelength, high-speed SS-OCT (~1,050 nm) OCTA was shown to have improved visualization of CNV compared to a shorter-wavelength (~840 nm), commercially available SD-OCT device.[11] In another study using the same SS-OCT prototype, SS-OCTA images of the choriocapillaris underlying drusen showed improved visualization as compared to the shorter wavelength SD-OCTA images.[45]

18.2 Advances in Optical Coherence Tomography Angiography Algorithms

The OCT signal contains both amplitude and phase components, and angiography methods can be based on the amplitude, phase, or the complex signal, which is a combination of both amplitude and phase information.[12] There are several software-based angiography techniques. An OCTA method that calculates speckle variance was reported by Mariampillai et al.[13] More recently, Jia et al described split-spectrum amplitude-decorrelation angiography (SSADA), which splits the spectrum into multiple smaller bands, resulting in improved signal-to-noise ratio.[14]

The optical microangiography algorithm utilizes a combination of phase and magnitude information for a theoretical improvement in sensitivity.[12,15,16,17] Recently, Zhang et al proposed a novel feature space-based optical microangiography method (fsO-MAG) in which the flow and static background are differentiated in the feature space, leading to the suppression of angiographic signals from the static background.[18] Reisman et al also recently reported the OCT angiography ratio algorithm (OCTARA), which utilizes a ratio method that keeps the full spectrum intact which may preserve axial resolution[46]. The rapid expansion of OCTA may lead to further development of software-based angiography methods, as well as improvements on existing methods.

One additional challenge in the interpretation of OCTA is that projection artifacts can confound interpretation and affect quantification of vascular abnormalities. Zhang et al recently reported a projection-resolved OCTA algorithm that is able to generate OCTA images while minimizing projection artifact, resolving ambiguity between projection artifact and in situ flow.[19]

18.3 Quantitative Analysis of Optical Coherence Tomography Angiography

OCTA enables rapid, noninvasive visualization of the retinal and choroidal vasculature. It can be easily performed at multiple follow-ups, making it a promising tool for monitoring the progression of disease and guiding treatment decisions. Algorithms for analyzing vessel density and assessing ischemia have been reported in diseases such as diabetic retinopathy (DR), where ischemia has been associated with worse visual outcomes.[20,21,22] These studies have demonstrated increased ischemia in DR and other vascular diseases and correlated ischemia with worse visual outcomes. To date, multiple novel algorithms have been applied to eyes with DR to quantify the ratio between areas of flow and areas of flow impairment.[23,24]

Jia et al have described a quantitative flow index that was applied to a prototype SS-OCT dataset, enabling the quantification of blood flow in CNV, optic disc perfusion in glaucoma, and other vascular abnormalities.[25,26,27] Chu et al proposed a five-index quantitative analysis of OCT angiograms, which includes vessel area density, vessel skeleton density, vessel diameter index, vessel perimeter index, and vessel complexity index. This represents a tool that can be used to quantify multiple features of vasculature on OCTA that represents a rapid strategy for interpreting OCT angiograms from multiple perspectives.[28] Moving forward, it is also important to consider the utility of these automated algorithms in real-life clinical datasets and normal patients, which include motion artifact and noise, which can affect accurate analysis. Larger studies are needed to validate these methods, as these may represent potential clinical endpoints on OCTA that can be used as biomarkers for future clinical trials.

A limitation of OCTA imaging is that the images of the vasculature provide limited information on the speed of flow in vessels. Variable interscan time analysis (VISTA), proposed by Choi and Moult et al,[29] is a tool that has been used to differentiate blood flow speeds on OCTA. High-speed systems are able to acquire multiple sequential OCT B-scans at the same location. These sequentially acquired OCT B-scans can then be analyzed with variable interscan time between the pairs. By varying the interscan time, different ranges of blood flow speeds can be visualized.[29] The VISTA analysis can be visualized using color coding (▶ Fig. 18.1 and ▶ Fig. 18.2) in which the color of the pixel represents the erythrocyte flow at a given location. The hue value of each VISTA pixel is a ratio of the OCTA signal obtained from the 1.5-ms interscan time to the OCTA signal from the 3-ms interscan time. In this case, blue pixels indicate slower speeds and red pixels indicate faster speeds.[47]

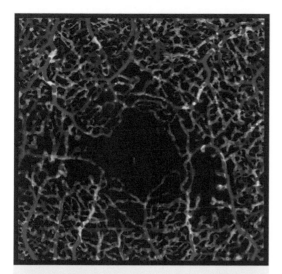

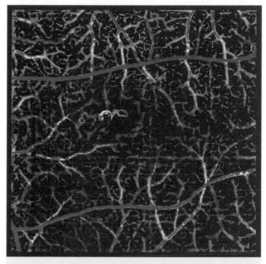

Fig. 18.1 Variable interscan time analysis (VISTA) visualization applied to a 3 × 3 mm optical coherence tomography angiography image from a patient with nonproliferative diabetic retinopathy. In this image, flow speeds of the vasculature in the superficial plexus are visualized using a color-encoded images in which red represents relatively high flow and blue represents areas of relatively low flow. Imaging was performed using a prototype ultrahigh-speed swept-source optical coherence tomography device developed at Massachusetts Institute of Technology. The device uses a 1,050-nm vertical-cavity surface-emitting laser (VCSEL) swept light source with a 400-kHz A-scan rate.

Fig. 18.2 Variable interscan time analysis (VISTA) visualization applied to a 3 × 3 mm optical coherence tomography angiography image from a patient with choroidal neovascularization secondary to age-related macular degeneration who had been previously treated with multiple intravitreal injections of anti–vascular endothelial growth factor. In this image, flow speeds of the vasculature in the superficial plexus are visualized using a color-encoded images in which red represents relatively high flow and blue represents areas of relatively low flow. Lower flow vessels (blue and green) can be seen at the periphery of the neovascular membrane, with a central area of relatively higher flow (yellow and red vessels). Imaging was performed using a prototype ultrahigh-speed swept-source optical coherence tomography device developed at Massachusetts Institute of Technology. The device uses a 1,050-nm vertical-cavity surface-emitting laser (VCSEL) swept light source with a 400-kHz A-scan rate.

18.4 Quantifying Ocular Blood Flow with Doppler Optical Coherence Tomography

OCTA has its origins in Doppler OCT techniques.[30,31,32,33] These techniques can be applied to traditional OCT imaging. While this is not a specific application of OCTA, it represents a relatively novel application of an existing technology that can quantitatively assess blood flow.

The principle behind Doppler-based imaging techniques is measuring the Doppler frequency shift of reflected light from the moving blood cells, and calculating blood flow velocity based on this information. In vivo measurement of retinal blood flow have been performed using multiple techniques including bidirectional laser Doppler velocimetry, scanning laser Doppler flowmetry, ultrasound color Doppler imaging, and both time- and Fourier-domain OCT. In laser Doppler velocimetry, each retinal vessel is measured individually, resulting in long scanning times. Scanning laser flowmetry is faster, but can only detect Doppler velocity in one direction. The limited resolution of ultrasound color Doppler imaging is insufficient to visualize the blood vessels in order to calculate the cross-sectional area, but can detect flow velocity in the ophthalmic artery at greater depths.[34,35,36,37,38]

Fourier-domain OCT utilizes optical phase information to precisely measure Doppler velocity.[34] It measures the axial flow velocity, which is the velocity component in the direction of the OCT probe beam. It provides quantitative measurement of high flow velocities in the retinal vessels of the optic disc, and is done by scanning multiple concentric circles around the optic disc. This technique requires the measurement of the Doppler angle between the velocity vector and the OCT probe beam, which is susceptible to errors and limits the automation of this particular Doppler OCT technique.[39,40,41]

Recently, high-speed, Fourier-domain en face Doppler OCT has been developed, which is a volumetric imaging method in which total blood flow (TRBF) is calculated in the plane orthogonal to the OCT probe beam. It measures TRBF by scanning a small area at the optic disc and integrating the axial blood flow velocity in the central retinal artery.[42,43,44] It does not require calculation of the Doppler angle, which allows for a fully automated calculation of TRBF. This technique has been performed on prototype systems only, and is not currently commercially available.

This technique has been used to investigate TRBF in several ocular diseases, including DR, retinal vein occlusions, uveitis, and glaucoma. In eyes with vein occlusions, the TRBF was reduced in the eye with the vascular occlusion, when compared to both the fellow eye and the normal age-matched eyes. In eyes with DR, TRBF is reduced in eyes with diabetic macular edema (DME) compared to those without DME. There was a significant reduction in TRBF in eyes with both active and existing uveitis compared to normal subjects. Interestingly, patients with active uveitis had further decrease on TRBF compared to inactive uveitis.[45] The findings of Jia et al suggested that in early glaucoma the reduction of optic nerve head (ONH) microvascular flow is much more dramatic than that of whole ONH circulation.[27]

Alterations in retinal blood flow are associated with the development of ocular diseases, and the development of Doppler OCT is a promising new technique for quantitative assessment of total retinal blood flow. Future, large-scale clinical studies may validate retinal blood flow as a diagnostic marker or utilize these measurements to inform treatment decisions.

18.5 Conclusion

In recent years, OCTA has rapidly expanded as an imaging modality that has been used to qualitatively and quantitatively describe changes in retinal and choroidal vasculature–associated pathology. It also has the potential to enhance our understanding of the disease mechanism, since microvascular changes can be correlated to structural features. Currently, OCTA is not widely used in the clinical setting to guide treatment or diagnosis decisions; however, it represents a promising modality for both clinical

decision-making as well as evaluating endpoints that can be used in clinical trials. Improvements in the hardware and software components of OCTA, as well as a standardized interpretation of these images and their artifacts by ophthalmologists are important for the further development of this imaging modality.

References

[1] Saito M, Iida T, Nagayama D. Cross-sectional and en face optical coherence tomographic features of polypoidal choroidal vasculopathy. Retina. 2008; 28(3):459–464

[2] Ueno C, Gomi F, Sawa M, Nishida K. Correlation of indocyanine green angiography and optical coherence tomography findings after intravitreal ranibizumab for polypoidal choroidal vasculopathy. Retina. 2012; 32(10):2006–2013

[3] Povazay B, Hermann B, Unterhuber A, et al. Three-dimensional optical coherence tomography at 1050 nm versus 800 nm in retinal pathologies: enhanced performance and choroidal penetration in cataract patients. J Biomed Opt. 2007; 12(4):041211

[4] Unterhuber A, Povazay B, Hermann B, Sattmann H, Chavez-Pirson A, Drexler W. In vivo retinal optical coherence tomography at 1040 nm - enhanced penetration into the choroid. Opt Express. 2005; 13(9):3252–3258

[5] Chinn SR, Swanson EA, Fujimoto JG. Optical coherence tomography using a frequency-tunable optical source. Opt Lett. 1997; 22(5):340–342

[6] An L, Wang RK. In vivo volumetric imaging of vascular perfusion within human retina and choroids with optical micro-angiography. Opt Express. 2008; 16(15):11438–11452

[7] Yasuno Y, Hong Y, Makita S, et al. In vivo high-contrast imaging of deep posterior eye by 1-micron swept source optical coherence tomography and scattering optical coherence angiography. Opt Express. 2007; 15(10):6121–6139

[8] Yasuno Y, Madjarova VD, Makita S, et al. Three-dimensional and high-speed swept-source optical coherence tomography for in vivo investigation of human anterior eye segments. Opt Express. 2005; 13(26):10652–10664

[9] Choma M, Sarunic M, Yang C, Izatt J. Sensitivity advantage of swept source and Fourier domain optical coherence tomography. Opt Express. 2003; 11(18):2183–2189

[10] Tatham, AJ. New swept-source OCT for glaucoma: improvements and advantages. Review of Ophthalmology. 2014. https://www.reviewofophthalmology.com/CMSDocuments-/2014/3/rp0314_topconi.pdf. Accessed on 12 April 2017

[11] Novais EA, Adhi M, Moult EM, et al. Choroidal neovascularization analyzed on ultrahigh-speed swept-source optical coherence tomography angiography compared to spectral-domain optical coherence tomography angiography. Am J Ophthalmol. 2016; 164:80–88

[12] Zhang A, Zhang Q, Chen CL, Wang RK. Methods and algorithms for optical coherence tomography-based angiography: a review and comparison. J Biomed Opt. 2015; 20(10):100901

[13] Mariampillai A, Standish BA, Moriyama EH, et al. Speckle variance detection of microvasculature using swept-source optical coherence tomography. Opt Lett. 2008; 33(13):1530–1532

[14] Jia Y, Tan O, Tokayer J, et al. Split-spectrum amplitude-decorrelation angiography with optical coherence tomography. Opt Express. 2012; 20(4):4710–4725

[15] Zhi Z, Chao JR, Wietecha T, Hudkins KL, Alpers CE, Wang RK. Noninvasive imaging of retinal morphology and microvasculature in obese mice using optical coherence tomography and optical microangiography. Invest Ophthalmol Vis Sci. 2014; 55(2):1024–1030

[16] Wang RK, An L, Francis P, Wilson DJ. Depth-resolved imaging of capillary networks in retina and choroid using ultrahigh sensitive optical microangiography. Opt Lett. 2010; 35(9): 1467–1469

[17] Wang RK, An L, Saunders S, Wilson DJ. Optical microangiography provides depth-resolved images of directional ocular blood perfusion in posterior eye segment. J Biomed Opt. 2010; 15(2):020502

[18] Zhang A, Wang RK. Feature space optical coherence tomography based micro-angiography. Biomed Opt Express. 2015; 6(5):1919–1928

[19] Zhang M, Hwang TS, Campbell JP, et al. Projection-resolved optical coherence tomographic angiography. Biomed Opt Express. 2016; 7(3):816–828

[20] Agemy SA, Scripsema NK, Shah CM, et al. Retinal vascular perfusion density mapping using optical coherence tomography angiography in normals and diabetic retinopathy patients. Retina. 2015; 35(11):2353–2363

[21] Hwang TS, Gao SS, Liu L, et al. Automated quantification of capillary nonperfusion using optical coherence tomography angiography in diabetic retinopathy. JAMA Ophthalmol. 2016; 134(4):367–373

[22] Lupidi M, Coscas F, Cagini C, et al. Automated quantitative analysis of retinal microvasculature in normal eyes on optical coherence tomography angiography. Am J Ophthalmol. 2016; 169:9–23

[23] Kim AY, Chu Z, Shahidzadeh A, Wang RK, Puliafito CA, Kashani AH. Quantifying microvascular density and morphology in diabetic retinopathy using spectral-domain optical coherence tomography angiography. Invest Ophthalmol Vis Sci. 2016; 57(9):OCT362–OCT370

[24] Schottenhamml J, Moult EM, Ploner S, et al. An automatic, intercapillary area-based algorithm for quantifying diabetes-related capillary dropout using optical coherence tomography angiography. Retina. 2016; 36 Suppl 1:S93–S101

[25] Jia Y, Bailey ST, Wilson DJ, et al. Quantitative optical coherence tomography angiography of choroidal neovascularization in age-related macular degeneration. Ophthalmology. 2014; 121(7):1435–1444

[26] Jia Y, Bailey ST, Hwang TS, et al. Quantitative optical coherence tomography angiography of vascular abnormalities in the living human eye. Proc Natl Acad Sci USA. 2015; 112(18):E2395–E2402

[27] Jia Y, Morrison JC, Tokayer J, et al. Quantitative OCT angiography of optic nerve head blood flow. Biomed Opt Express. 2012; 3(12):3127–3137

[28] Chu Z, Lin J, Gao C, et al. Quantitative assessment of the retinal microvasculature using optical coherence tomography angiography. J Biomed Opt. 2016; 21(6):66008

[29] Choi W, Moult EM, Waheed NK, et al. Ultrahigh-speed, swept-source optical coherence tomography angiography in nonexudative age-related macular degeneration with geographic atrophy. Ophthalmology. 2015; 122(12):2532–2544

[30] Makita S, Fabritius T, Yasuno Y. Quantitative retinal-blood flow measurement with three-dimensional vessel geometry determination using ultrahigh-resolution Doppler optical coherence angiography. Opt Lett. 2008; 33(8):836–838

[31] Makita S, Jaillon F, Yamanari M, Miura M, Yasuno Y. Comprehensive in vivo micro-vascular imaging of the human eye by dual-beam-scan Doppler optical coherence angiography. Opt Express. 2011; 19(2):1271–1283

[32] Wang RK, Jacques SL, Ma Z, Hurst S, Hanson SR, Gruber A. Three dimensional optical angiography. Opt Express. 2007; 15(7):4083–4097

[33] Wang RK. Three-dimensional optical micro-angiography maps directional blood perfusion deep within microcirculation tissue beds in vivo. Phys Med Biol. 2007; 52(23):N531–N537

[34] Leitgeb RA, Werkmeister RM, Blatter C, Schmetterer L. Doppler optical coherence tomography. Prog Retin Eye Res. 2014; 41:26–43

[35] Yu L, Chen Z. Doppler variance imaging for three-dimensional retina and choroid angiography. J Biomed Opt. 2010; 15(1):016029

[36] Makita S, Jaillon F, Yamanari M, Yasuno Y. Dual-beam-scan Doppler optical coherence angiography for birefringence-artifact-free vasculature imaging. Opt Express. 2012; 20(3): 2681–2692

[37] Grunwald JE, Riva CE, Sinclair SH, Brucker AJ, Petrig BL. Laser Doppler velocimetry study of retinal circulation in diabetes mellitus. Arch Ophthalmol. 1986; 104(7):991–996

[38] Lee JC, Wong BJ, Tan O, et al. Pilot study of Doppler optical coherence tomography of retinal blood flow following laser photocoagulation in poorly controlled diabetic patients. Invest Ophthalmol Vis Sci. 2013; 54(9):6104–6111

[39] Wang Y, Bower BA, Izatt JA, Tan O, Huang D. In vivo total retinal blood flow measurement by Fourier domain Doppler optical coherence tomography. J Biomed Opt. 2007; 12(4): 041215

[40] Wang Y, Bower BA, Izatt JA, Tan O, Huang D. Retinal blood flow measurement by circumpapillary Fourier domain Doppler optical coherence tomography. J Biomed Opt. 2008; 13(6):064003

[41] Wang Y, Lu A, Gil-Flamer J, Tan O, Izatt JA, Huang D. Measurement of total blood flow in the normal human retina using Doppler Fourier-domain optical coherence tomography. Br J Ophthalmol. 2009; 93(5):634–637

[42] Baumann B, Potsaid B, Kraus MF, et al. Total retinal blood flow measurement with ultrahigh speed swept source/Fourier domain OCT. Biomed Opt Express. 2011; 2(6):1539–1552

[43] Choi W, Baumann B, Liu JJ, et al. Measurement of pulsatile total blood flow in the human and rat retina with ultrahigh speed spectral/Fourier domain OCT. Biomed Opt Express. 2012; 3(5):1047–1061

[44] Choi W, Potsaid B, Jayaraman V, et al. Phase-sensitive swept-source optical coherence tomography imaging of the human retina with a vertical cavity surface-emitting laser light source. Opt Lett. 2013; 38(3):338–340

[45] Lane M, Moult EM, Novais EA, et al. Visualizing the Choriocapillaris under Drusen: Comparing 1050-nm swept-source versus 840-nm spectral-domain optical coherence tomography angiography. Investigative Ophthalmology and Visual Science. 2016; 57(9):585–590

[46] Reisman, et al. IOVS 2016;43:ARVO E-Abstract 452

[47] Ploner SB, Moult EM, Choi W, et al. Toward quantitative optical coherence tomography angiography: Visualizing blood flow speeds in ocular pathology using variable interscan time analysis. Retina. 2016; 36 Suppl 1:S118–S126

19 Optical Coherence Tomography Angiography Rounds

David R. Chow

19.1 Case 1

A 68-year-old woman with a history of dry age-related macular degeneration (ARMD) and geographic atrophy OU presented to the office complaining of some distortion in her left eye (▶ Fig. 19.1). The visual acuity was 20/50 OD and 20/40 OS. On examination, there was a patch of geographic atrophy (GA) involving the nasal and superior macula (▶ Fig. 19.1a). There was a dot hemorrhage located just superotemporal to the fovea just inferior to the edge of clinically evident GA. Early-phase fluorescein angiography (FA) revealed a window defect in the area of GA (▶ Fig. 19.1b). Late-phase FA revealed a small area of hyperfluorescence in the direct area of the retinal hemorrhage seen clinically consistent with a neovascular membrane or retinal angiomatous

proliferation (RAP) lesion (▶ Fig. 19.1c). Optical coherence tomography (OCT) angiogram of superficial retina plexus reveals a focal area of increased signal corresponding to the area of retinal hemorrhage consistent with type 3 choroidal neovascular membrane (CNVM) or RAP lesion (▶ Fig. 19.1d). OCT angiogram of deep retinal plexus reveals the same area of increased signal corresponding to the area of retinal hemorrhage consistent with type 3 CNVM or RAP lesion (▶ Fig. 19.1e). OCT angiogram of outer retina revealed a focal decorrelation signal corresponding to the area of retinal hemorrhage consistent with type 3 CNVM or RAP lesion extending into outer retina (▶ Fig. 19.1f). The structural OCT shows the presence of intraretinal fluid (inset). OCT angiogram of choroid choriocapillaris shows projection artifact of superficial retinal plexus onto choroidal image (▶ Fig. 19.1g).

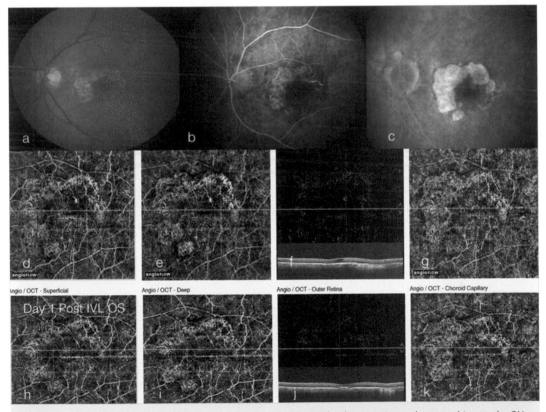

Fig. 19.1 A 68-year-old woman with a history of dry age-related macular degeneration and geographic atrophy OU presented to the office complaining of some distortion in her left eye. The visual acuity was 20/50 OD and 20/40 OS. *(continued)*

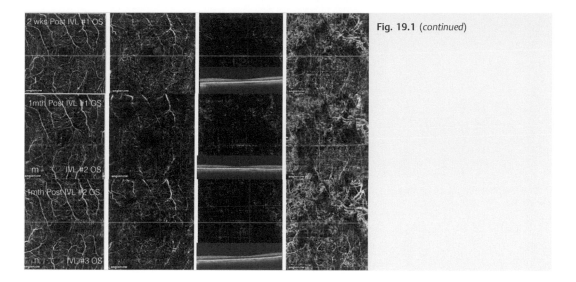

Fig. 19.1 (*continued*)

The initial assessment of the patients imaging allowed us to confirm the presence of wet ARMD OS. The OCT angiogram provided information we would not have had from the FA alone by allowing us to determine the neovascular membrane originated in the retina itself consistent with a type 3 CNVM or RAP lesion. The OCT angiogram in this patient also highlights the difficulties related to projection artifacts confusing the images obtained in other slabs. Based on the images obtained, a decision was made to proceed with anti–vascular endothelial growth factor (anti-VEGF) therapy OS.

Day 1 post-injection of intravitreal Lucentis (IVL) OS, OCT angiogram of the superficial and deep retinal plexus shows the RAP lesion has disappeared (▶ Fig. 19.1h, i). OCT angiogram of the outer retina shows disappearance of the RAP lesion and the inset structural OCT scan shows the intraretinal fluid has resolved as well (▶ Fig. 19.1j). OCT angiogram choroid choriocapillaris shows projection artifact of the superficial retina but no CNVM (▶ Fig. 19.1k). Two weeks post-IVL number 1 OS, the patient returned for another OCT angiogram and this scan continued to show no evidence of the RAP lesion and no fluid on the structural OCT (▶ Fig. 19.1l). One month post-injection, the patient returned for her second IVL OS (▶ Fig. 19.1m). The OCT angiogram at this visit did not show any evidence of recurrence of the RAP lesion or fluid on the structural OCT. One month post-injection number 2, the patient returned for her third IVL OS (▶ Fig. 19.1n). The OCT angiogram at this visit did not show any evidence of recurrence of the RAP lesion or fluid on the structural OCT.

The serial usage of OCT angiograms in this patient was able to elegantly show the positive response to the initial injection of intravitreal anti-VEGF therapy with regression of the RAP lesion within 24 hours. Given OCT angiograms are noninvasive, they can be performed frequently and may become very useful in gauging a patient's response to therapy. During the patient's monthly visits, there was no evidence of reperfusion of the RAP lesion at 1-month visits. This may be clinically valuable to determine at what interval a patient can get away without maintenance therapy.

19.2 Case 2

A 79-year-old woman presented with a history of mild dry ARMD OU (▶ Fig. 19.2). She had no visual complaints on presentation. Her visual acuity was OD 20/100 OS 20/80. The fundus examination revealed some stippled RPE pigmentary changes but no blood or obvious fluid OD (▶ Fig. 19.2a). The fundus examination OS revealed mild drusen and RPE changes (▶ Fig. 19.2b). The structural OCT OD revealed some subretinal fluid and intraretinal fluid (▶ Fig. 19.2c). The structural OCT OS revealed mild drusen (▶ Fig. 19.2d). The fluorescein angiogram early-phase OD showed a central RPE perfusion defect (▶ Fig. 19.2e). The mid-phase fluorescein angiogram OD showed stippled hyperfluorescence on the temporal border of the overt lesion (▶ Fig. 19.2f). The late-phase fluorescein angiogram OD showed progressive stippled hyperfluorescence now covering the entire lesion (▶ Fig. 19.2g). The OCT angiogram showed no overt changes in the

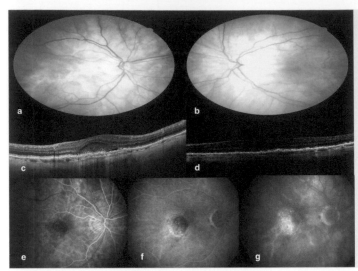

Fig. 19.2 A 79-year-old woman presented with a history of mild dry age-related macular degeneration OU. She had no visual complaints on presentation. Her visual acuity was OD 20/100 OS 20/80. (*continued*)

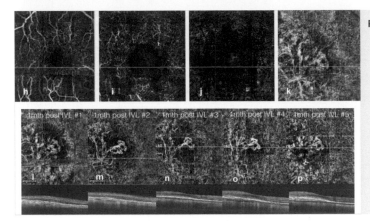

Fig. 19.2 (*continued*)

superficial (▶ Fig. 19.2h) and deep (▶ Fig. 19.2i) retinal plexus, nor in the outer retina (▶ Fig. 19.2j), but did show an obvious large CNVM in the choriocapillaris (▶ Fig. 19.2k) characterized by a central feeder vessel with a branching fan-shaped pattern emanating from the feeder vessel.

Based on the patient's initial multimodal imaging, a diagnosis of a type 1 occult CNVM from ARMD OD was made. Interestingly, the patient was asymptomatic at presentation, so a discussion was carried out about the nature of the pathology and risks of progression without treatment. The patient elected to commence anti-VEGF therapy with IVL.

One month post-IVL OD number 1, the structural OCT shows disappearance of the subretinal fluid and the OCT angiogram shows pruning of the peripheral new branches of the CNVM (▶ Fig. 19.2l). One month post-IVL OD number 2, the structural OCT is dry and the OCT angiogram shows an obvious drop in the perfusion of the CNVM complex

(▶ Fig. 19.2m). One month post-IVL number 3 and number 4, the structural OCT stays dry and the OCT angiogram shows a similar reduction in the perfusion of the CNVM complex to the previous months (▶ Fig. 19.2n, o). One month post-IVL number 5, the structural OCT stays dry and there is obvious remodeling of the CNVM complex on the OCT angiogram (▶ Fig. 19.2p).

The sequential OCT angiograms used on this patient with wet ARMD provide another piece of information to guide us in our decision-making. The current management of patients with wet ARMD is largely based on the presence or absence of fluid on structural OCT scans. OCT angiograms now allow us to monitor the perfusion of the CNVM complex in response to therapy. Other investigators have already noted different patterns of therapeutic response to treatment with anti-VEGF therapies. Some CNVM complexes entirely disappear on OCT angiograms following therapy only to reappear as therapy wears off, providing valuable insight into the recurrence patterns for a given patient. Unfortunately, in our experience, although we have noted some patients who do show dramatic responses to anti-VEGF therapy with disappearance of the CNVM complex, the majority of patients tend to show a partial response like this patient with pruning of the branches of the CNVM complex and persistent flow in the trunk or feeder vessel. Many investigators have noted this similar phenomenon. The value of monitoring the perfusion of the CNVM complex and using this to guide treatment decisions has yet to be validated in clinical trials. We will need to better study and understand the patterns of response in CNVM complexes to determine if there are certain characteristics of the complex or their response to therapy, which can be used to guide therapy or provide prognostic information.

19.3 Case 3

A 68-year-old woman who has been getting intravitreal injections in her left eye for 8 months presented to the clinic (► Fig. 19.3). Her visual acuity was 20/200. She was put on a treat-and-extend regimen after her initial loading dose with a recurrence of fluid on structural OCT at 6-week intervals. Eight months into her treatment, OCT angiography became available with sequential images then taken at each follow-up visit to help in the decision of the timing of her next treatment. The fundus photo at the time of her 8-month visit with an obvious choroidal neovascular membrane is seen on exam with no obvious hemorrhage

(► Fig. 19.3a). The structural OCT insert shows intraretinal fluid and a sub-RPE lesion at 6 weeks post-injection. As a result of the fluid on her structural OCT, she was asked to return at 4 weeks for her next injection. The OCT angiogram at this visit shows the CNVM complex in the choriocapillaris with an obvious sea fan configuration and a dry structural OCT (► Fig. 19.3b). Since the structural OCT was dry, she was extended to 5 weeks. OCT angiography at this visit showed what appeared to be increased perfusion of the CNVM complex with the same surface area and a dry structural OCT (► Fig. 19.3c). The interesting question arising from these images is, do we as clinicians stick to our trial-tested indications for treatment (structural OCT fluid) or do we take into account the new OCT angiogram image showing what appears to be increasing perfusion of the CNVM complex at a 5-week interval. A decision was made to have the patient return again at 4 weeks instead of 5 due to the concerns related to the presumed increasing perfusion of the CNVM complex at a 5-week interval. This decision was based on a presumption that increasing perfusion of the CNVM complex would likely precede the development of fluid in the retina and that comparing sequential images of the perfusion of the CNVM complex might allow clinicians to institute therapy at an earlier stage before fluid develops in the retina. This presumption, of course, is not validated in any clinical trials at this point and may be entirely wrong or only applicable in certain situations the characteristics of which have yet to be determined. Four weeks later, the patient returned for her next

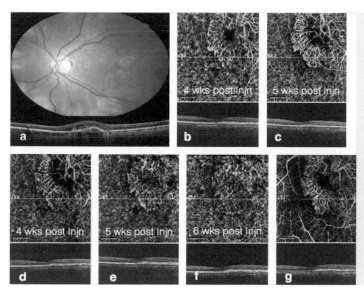

Fig. 19.3 A 68-year-old woman who has been getting intravitreal injections in her left eye for 8 months. Her visual acuity was 20/200. She was put on a treat-and-extend regimen after her initial loading dose with a recurrence of fluid on structural optical coherence tomography (OCT) at 6-week intervals. Eight months into her treatment, OCT angiography became available with sequential images then taken at each follow-up visit to help in the decision of the timing of her next treatment.

injection with an OCT angiogram showing what appears to be a marked reduction in perfusion with some obvious pruning of the sea fan vessels (▶ Fig. 19.3d). The structural OCT was dry. Based on the images, a decision was made to extend her next visit to 5 weeks. Five weeks later, the OCT angiogram showed what appeared to be a further reduction in perfusion with further pruning of vessels in the sea fan and a dry structural OCT again (▶ Fig. 19.3e). Based on these images, a decision was made to try and extend the interval to 6 weeks. Six weeks later, the OCT angiogram showed what appeared to be a significant reduction in perfusion of the CNVM complex with a dry structural OCT (▶ Fig. 19.3f). Given some skepticism about the dramatic improvement of the CNVM complex, the images were reviewed again; however, this time with manual segmentation. After manually segmented, the perfusion and surface area of the CNVM complex looked similar to that done 6 weeks previously (▶ Fig. 19.3g). The lesson learned from these images is extremely important for clinicians to realize particularly if you are going to try and sequentially compare the perfusion and surface area of CNVM complexes. Do not forget that each image obtained on a patient has autosegmentation software applied to it and that from visit to visit the registration of each slab you are looking at is not necessarily exactly the same. This is critically important so that you do not make treatment decisions based on the progression analysis of OCT angiogram images, which may not represent exactly the same slab. The importance of giving clinicians comparable images over time has not been lost on the manufacturers of OCT machines, all of whom are addressing this current problem. The ability to monitor the actual perfusion and size of CNVM complexes through therapy is an exciting opportunity that OCT angiography offers us that will be thoroughly studied over the next few years.

19.4 Case 4

A 68-year-old male presented with some distortion in his left eye. His visual acuity was 20/50 (▶ Fig. 19.4). The clinical examination revealed numerous soft drusen with central coalescence into a drusenoid pigment epithelial detachment (PED; ▶ Fig. 19.4a). The structural OCT revealed a drusenoid PED but also some subretinal fluid (▶ Fig. 19.4d). As a result, a fluorescein angiogram was ordered. The early-phase (▶ Fig. 19.4b) and late-phase (▶ Fig. 19.4c) fluorescein angiogram did not reveal any overt CNVM. An OCT angiogram was ordered and interestingly a CNVM was identified in the choriocapillaris directly beneath the drusenoid PED with some projection artifacts as well (▶ Fig. 19.4e). This is one of a growing group of anecdotal cases where OCT angiography allows a CNVM to be identified, which was missed on traditional FA. Publications have already noted the ability of OCT angiography to identify CNVM in patients with chronic central serous chorioretinopathy, where traditional FA reveals indeterminate leakage. This capability has also been identified in patients with CNVM secondary to uveitis. This case is a little different in that in the two previous situations fluorescein leakage from the original condition "masks" the CNVM, which then develops, whereas in this case there is NO fluorescein leakage or it is masked by the drusenoid PED. There are a number of series of similar patients now being put together for publication.

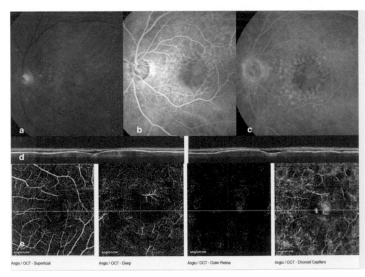

Fig. 19.4 A 68-year-old male presented with some distortion in his left eye. His visual acuity was 20/50.

19.5 Case 5

An 85-year-old male with a history of dry ARMD presented for routine follow-up examination (▶ Fig. 19.5). He was asymptomatic on presentation. The clinical examination revealed scattered soft drusen OU with no overt retinal hemorrhage (▶ Fig. 19.5a). The structural OCT revealed some subretinal fluid (▶ Fig. 19.5d). As a result, a fluorescein angiogram was ordered. The early-phase fluorescein angiogram (▶ Fig. 19.5b) revealed subtle mild hyperfluorescence inferonasal to the fovea and the late phase (▶ Fig. 19.5c) confirmed mild progressive hyperfluorescence consistent with a type 1 occult CNVM. An OCT angiogram was performed that revealed an obvious type 1 CNVM complex in the choriocapillaris (▶ Fig. 19.5e). Because the patient was asymptomatic, he elected not to receive any therapy. As a result, we followed the patient monthly for signs of progression. Over the next 6 months, there was obvious growth of the CNVM complex on OCT angiography with a slight increase in the amount of subretinal fluid on structural OCT (▶ Fig. 19.5f–k). Throughout this time period, the patient remained asymptomatic and despite many conversations about the concerns related to just monitoring his condition, he preferred to be observed. At last follow-up, he continues to remain asymptomatic. This patient beautifully illustrates the value of serial OCT angiograms to monitor the evolution of a CNVM complex in asymptomatic patients. The OCT angiograms offer more value in the follow-up of this patient than do the structural OCT scans.

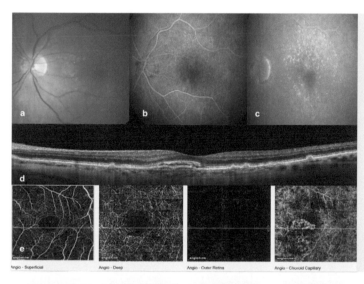

Fig. 19.5 An 85-year-old male with a history of dry age-related macular degeneration presents for routine follow-up examination. He was asymptomatic on presentation. (*continued*)

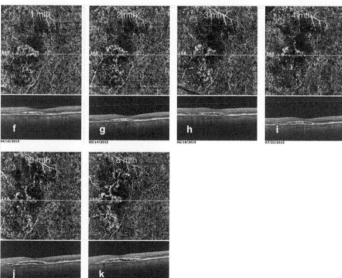

Fig. 19.5 (*continued*)

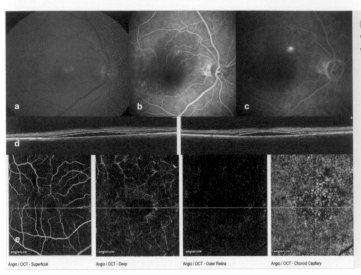

Fig. 19.6 A 33-year-old male presents with a 2-month history of reduced vision OD to 20/80.

Angio / OCT - Superficial   Angio / OCT - Deep   Angio / OCT - Outer Retina   Angio / OCT - Choroid Capillary

19.6 Case 6

A 33-year-old male presented with a 2-month history of reduced vision OD to 20/80 (▶ Fig. 19.6). The clinical examination revealed a serous detachment of the macula in a vertical oblong configuration (▶ Fig. 19.6a). The structural OCT scan confirmed the serous detachment of the retina (▶ Fig. 19.6d, e). A fluorescein angiogram was performed, which revealed a pinpoint leak in the superior macula in the early phase (▶ Fig. 19.6b) with progressive leakage from these pinpoint foci in the late phase (▶ Fig. 19.6c) of the angiogram. An OCT angiogram was performed, which revealed a speckled pattern of hyperperfusion surrounded by areas of hypoperfusion in the choriocapillaris in the body of the serous detachment. A clinical diagnosis of acute central serous chorioretinopathy (CSC) was made with a single pinpoint leak. OCT angiography can be very helpful in cases of presumed CSC given it has a distinctive pattern of speckled hyperperfusion around areas of hypoperfusion in the choriocapillaris. This pattern of perfusion is usually limited to the body of the serous retinal detachment. A number of early investigators have made similar observations. There is some question and argument, however, about whether these changes persist on resolution of the serous retinal detachment and whether these changes respond to therapy. The findings on OCT angiography have been found to nicely mimic those seen on indocyanine green (ICG) angiography.

19.7 Case 7

A 45-year-old with high myope (−8D OU) presented with some distortion and blurred vision OD (▶ Fig. 19.7). The clinical examination revealed a typical fundus for a high myope with a myopic disc, angulation of the vessels, myopic macular degenerative changes, lacquer cracks, and, of recent importance, a retinal hemorrhage in the temporal macula adjacent to a lacquer crack (▶ Fig. 19.7a). The structural OCT scan revealed (▶ Fig. 19.7b) a small focus of a myopic CNVM with no overt associated retinal fluid adjacent to the (▶ Fig. 19.7c) lacquer crack, which had an obvious break in Bruch's membrane with associated choroidal excavation. A fluorescein angiogram was ordered, which revealed in the early (▶ Fig. 19.7d) and mid stages (▶ Fig. 19.7e) a small focus of mild hyperfluorescence adjacent to the blockage from the retinal hemorrhage. In the late stages of the angiogram (▶ Fig. 19.7f), there was mild hyperfluorescent leakage emanating from the area adjacent to the retinal hemorrhage. Given the clinical features, structural OCT, and fluorescein angiogram, a diagnosis of myopic CNVM was made OD. A 3 × 3 mm OCT angiogram was ordered, which revealed increased visibility of the larger choroidal vessels but no overt CNVM in the choriocapillaris slab (▶ Fig. 19.7g). A 6 × 6 mm OCT angiogram was performed, which revealed the myopic CNVM as small focal area of hyperperfusion correlating with the site of leakage on FA and the structural OCT showing the small elevation of the RPE

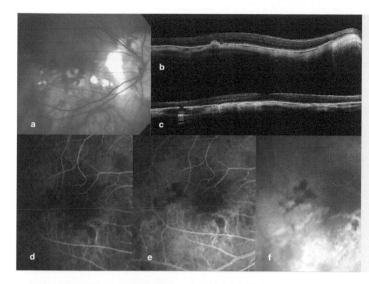

Fig. 19.7 A 45-year-old with high myope (−8D OU) presented with some distortion and blurred vision OD. (*continued*)

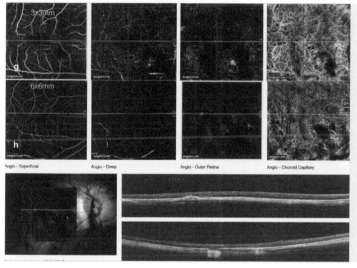

Fig. 19.7 (*continued*)

(▶ Fig. 19.7h). These two OCT angiograms nicely illustrate that although the standard 3 × 3 mm scans have higher resolution than the 6 × 6 mm scans, they are of course limited in their scope to catch pathology outside the central 3 × 3 mm unless you train your technician to take the 3 × 3 mm scan eccentrically. There is hope as technology improves that the resolution seen with the 3 × 3 mm scans can be translated into larger scanning areas.

19.8 Case 8

A 52-year-old male with a history of type 2 diabetes mellitus for 12 years presented for routine follow-up exam after having had successful treatment for mild diabetic macular edema in both eyes with light focal laser (▶ Fig. 19.8). The clinical exam showed neovascularization of the disc (NVD) less than one-third the disc diameter (▶ Fig. 19.8a). A fluorescein angiogram showed progressive hyperfluorescence of the NVD through the early (▶ Fig. 19.8b) mid (▶ Fig. 19.8c) and late (▶ Fig. 19.8d) phases of the angiogram with some microaneurysms scattered particularly through the temporal macula. The structural OCT of the optic nerve head (▶ Fig. 19.8e) showed the neovascular tissue above the optic nerve head. The fundus photo and fluorescein angiogram of the NVD were compared to the OCT angiogram of the optic nerve head (▶ Fig. 19.8f) focused on the vitreous,

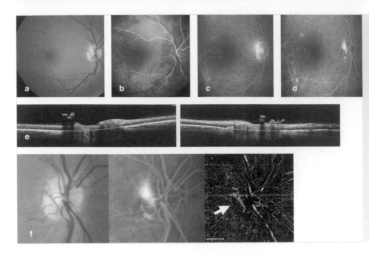

Fig. 19.8 A 52-year-old male with a history of type 2 diabetes mellitus for 12 years presented for routine follow-up exam after having had successful treatment for mild diabetic macular edema in both eyes with light focal laser. (*continued*)

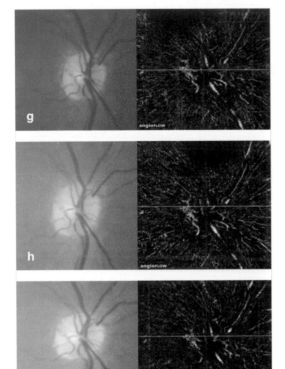

Fig. 19.8 (*continued*)

above the optic nerve. The OCT angiogram of the optic nerve head showed the anatomy of the neovascular tissue (white arrow) with more definition and clarity than the fluorescein angiogram. Based on the high-risk features of proliferative diabetic retinopathy (PDR) in this eye, a decision was made to progress to panretinal photocoagulation (PRP).

Two weeks following his first session of PRP laser, he returned for his second session and an OCT angiogram was performed (▶ Fig. 19.8g) to look for any changes in the perfusion or size of the neovascular tissue. At this visit, we were unconvinced of any particular change in these variables. He received his second PRP session of 180 degrees and then returned 2 weeks later for reassessment. The OCT angiogram at this visit (▶ Fig. 19.8h, i), once again, showed very little change in the perfusion or size of the neovascular tissue. Having completed a 360-degree PRP laser, the patient was asked to return in a month, where the OCT angiogram was repeated again. At this visit (▶ Fig. 19.8i), there appeared to be some reduction in the perfusion and size of the neovascular tissue, but it was subtle. Our experience has shown a variable response in the perfusion of the NV tissue in PDR to PRP therapy. In some cases, there appears to be complete regression with absence of perfusion, but in many there is only a partial response to PRP therapy with continued perfusion of the NV complex at what appears to be lower flow levels. Other investigators have made similar observations. OCT angiography now provides us with a noninvasive way to monitor patient responses to PRP laser therapy or to anti-VEGF therapy, as the results of Protocol S are integrated into day-to-day practice. We need to learn more about the patterns of response on OCT angiography to therapy in different patients with diabetes to help guide our decision-making.

19.9 Case 9

A 38-year-old patient with type 1 diabetes for 18 years who had been treated and followed up for

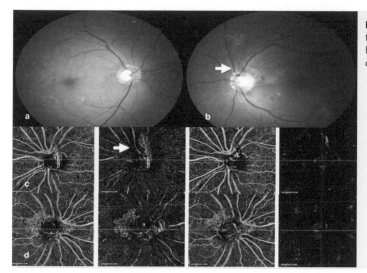

Fig. 19.9 A 38-year-old patient with type 1 diabetes for 18 years who had been treated and followed up for diabetic macular edema.

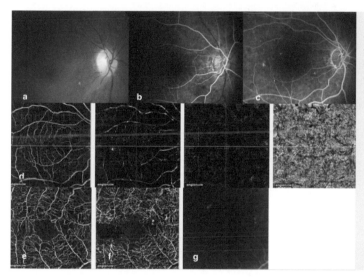

Fig. 19.10 A 54-year-old patient with type 2 diabetes for 15 years presents for a routine follow-up examination of diabetic retinopathy. The clinical examination revealed mild to moderate nonproliferative diabetic retinopathy OD.

diabetic macular edema presented to the clinic (▶ Fig. 19.9). On a routine follow-up visit, neovascularization of the disc was diagnosed OS on clinical examination (▶ Fig. 19.9b, arrow). At that same visit, the clinical examination of the disc OD (▶ Fig. 19.9a) failed to reveal any overt neovascularization. An OCT angiogram of the optic nerve was performed in both eyes. In the left eye (▶ Fig. 19.9c), there was a very obvious vertically oriented growth of new vessels in the vitreous above the optic nerve, which correlated to the NVD seen clinically in this eye (arrow). The OCT angiogram of the right eye, however, was a surprise as it revealed a very obvious growth of NVD around the optic nerve

(▶ Fig. 19.9d). This NVD OD had been missed clinically and on reexamining the patient, the flat details of this NVD so easily seen on OCT angiography were evident. This case nicely illustrates how OCT angiography of the optic nerve may become very useful in patients with diabetes to pick up NVD.

19.10 Case 10

A 54-year-old patient with type 2 diabetes for 15 years presented for a routine follow-up examination of diabetic retinopathy (▶ Fig. 19.10). The clinical examination revealed mild to moderate non-PDR OD (▶ Fig. 19.10a). There was no clinical or structural OCT evidence of macular edema. A fluorescein angiogram was done, which revealed scattered microaneurysms with mild leakage throughout the macula in the early (▶ Fig. 19.10b) and late (▶ Fig. 19.10c) phases of the angiogram. An OCT angiogram was performed, which revealed subtle poorly defined anomalies in the superficial and deep retinal plexus (▶ Fig. 19.10d). This OCT angiogram was performed at 8 × 8 mm. The OCT angiogram was repeated at 3 × 3 mm, which revealed in nice detail the anomalies typically seen in diabetic retinopathy. The superficial retina plexus (▶ Fig. 19.10e) revealed enlargement of the foveal avascular zone with focal areas of capillary nonperfusion and rarefaction of the capillaries. There were no overt microaneurysms noted. The deep retinal plexus (▶ Fig. 19.10f) revealed similar findings but greater enlargement of the foveal avascular zone and obvious microaneurysms. The findings on the OCT angiogram were compared to those found on the fluorescein angiogram (▶ Fig. 19.10g). Interestingly, the correlation between what was seen on the OCT angiogram in the superficial and deep retinal plexus was not identical to the microaneurysms seen on FA. In this patient, there were microaneurysms seen on FA, which were not evident in either the superficial or the deep retinal plexus. Other investigators have noted similar findings with some aneurysms showing up on OCT angiography that do not appear on traditional FA and vice versa. There is evolving work being done to correlate the vascular anomalies seen in the superficial versus deep retinal plexus to traditional clinical parameters.

Anecdotally in our experience, we have noted a predominance of pathology in patients being clinically treated for diabetic macular edema in the deep retinal plexus compared to the superficial retinal plexus, but this needs to be substantiated. This patient also nicely demonstrates how important it is to obtain 3 × 3 mm scans to obtain the maximum resolution to evaluate the retinal vasculature.

19.11 Case 11

A 73-year-old male with a history of hypertension presented with reduced vision OS for 2 months (▶ Fig. 19.11). His vision on presentation was 20/200 OS. The clinical examination (▶ Fig. 19.11a) revealed an obvious superior branch retinal vein occlusion OS with a moderate amount of intraretinal hemorrhage and obvious macular edema. The structural OCT (▶ Fig. 19.11b) confirmed the macular edema with significant retinal thickening, intraretinal fluid, and subretinal fluid. An 8 × 8 mm OCT angiogram was done at presentation, which revealed a segment of capillary nonperfusion in the superonasal macula just distal to the occlusion site. This was seen in the superficial retinal plexus (▶ Fig. 19.11c). The deep retinal plexus (▶ Fig. 19.11d) was difficult to evaluate due to artifacts from signal loss related to the intraretinal blood and autosegmentation difficulties due to the anomalous anatomy created by the significant retinal thickening seen on the structural OCT scan. The outer retina (▶ Fig. 19.11e) and choriocapillaris (▶ Fig. 19.11f) showed no overt abnormalities

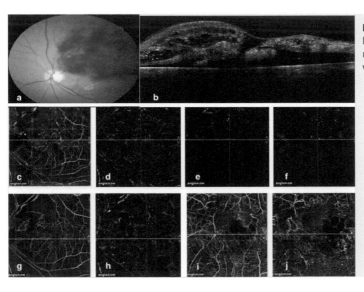

Fig. 19.11 A 73-year-old male with a history of hypertension presented with reduced vision OS for 2 months. His vision on presentation was 20/200 OS.

but did show signal loss due to the overlying blood. The patient was given an intravitreal injection of an anti-VEGF agent and returned 1 month later. The OCT angiogram at this visit was repeated at 8 × 8 mm and this showed a much more obvious area of capillary nonperfusion in the superonasal macula of the superficial retinal plexus (▶ Fig. 19.11g). The resolution of this image was greatly improved over the image at presentation due to the reduction in macula edema resulting in greater accuracy of the autosegmentation slab and the clearance of some of the intraretinal hemorrhage. The deep retinal plexus at this visit (▶ Fig. 19.11h) was still difficult to evaluate due to the signal loss from the intraretinal hemorrhage. At this visit, the OCT angiogram was repeated at 3 × 3 mm, with a significant improvement in resolution. The superficial retinal plexus at 3 × 3 mm (▶ Fig. 19.11i) showed multiple areas of capillary nonperfusion and anomalies of the capillary vasculature in the superior macula. The deep retinal plexus (▶ Fig. 19.11j) at 3 × 3 mm showed a significant improvement in resolution, allowing excellent evaluation of this retinal vascular plexus. On this image, there were similar findings to the superficial retinal plexus with large areas of capillary nonperfusion and vascular anomalies in the superior macula. Uniquely, this image revealed the intraretinal cysts, which were seen on this en face image as a cluster of oval black circles in the temporal macula. This case nicely illustrates the issues related to the sampling size in OCT angiography. To ideally evaluate patients with a retinal vein occlusion, we want a sample size that encompasses the entire macula. Although an 8 × 8 mm scan can provide enough width to encompass most of the pathology in retinal vein occlusions, the resolution is less than ideal to discern details. The 3 × 3 mm scan results in a significant increase in resolution but is unable to sample the whole area of pathology. In our practice, we have taken to performing both an 8 × 8 and a 3 × 3 mm scan in patients with retinal vein occlusions to try and capture the full pathology. Once again, there is promise for the future that the resolution on larger scan sizes will be improved through technological advances in the software and hardware of these imaging platforms.

Index

Note: Page numbers set **bold** or *italic* indicate headings or figures, respectively.